ENERGY BALANCE AND OBESITY IN MAN

Energy balance and obesity in man

2nd edition completely revised

J.S. GARROW

M.D.   Ph.D.   F.R.C.P.

Medical Research Council, Clinical Research Centre,
Watford Road, Harrow, England

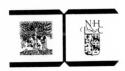

1978

ELSEVIER/NORTH-HOLLAND BIOMEDICAL PRESS
AMSTERDAM · NEW YORK · OXFORD

ISBN 0-444-80046-8

With 33 illustrations and 12 tables

Published by:

ELSEVIER/NORTH-HOLLAND BIOMEDICAL PRESS
335 Jan van Galenstraat
P.O. Box 211, Amsterdam, The Netherlands

Sole distributors for the U.S.A. and Canada:

ELSEVIER NORTH-HOLLAND, INC.
52 Vanderbilt Avenue
New York, New York 10017

First edition published in 1974

Library of Congress Cataloging in Publication Data

Garrow, J.S.
    Energy balance and obesity in man

    Bibliography: pp. 197–223
    Includes index.
    1.   Obesity.   2.   Energy   metabolism.   I.   Title.
RC628.G37   1978   616.3'98   78-2363
ISBN 0-444-80046-8

Printed in The Netherlands

To K.J.G.
now 1.72 m, 59 kg,
who still eats what
she likes

Acknowledgements

I am very grateful to all those who pointed out errors in the previous edition of this book or suggested improvements for this one, in particular G. Bray, J.V.G.A. Durnin, D. Lister, N. Norgan, R. Passmore and B.J. Stordy. It is not possible to name all the colleagues at the Clinical Research Centre who have helped me, but with the work described in this book the following have many times given advice, help or encouragement: D.G. Altman, Margaret Ashwell, J.A. Baker, G.M. Bull, R. Diethelm, Merril Durrant, D. Halliday, R. Hesp, M.J.R. Healy, Pat Hulme, S.J.E. Humphrey, Pat Poulter, Susan Stalley, Shirley Sunkin, Penelope Warwick, H.S. Wolff: it is delightful to work in such stimulating company.

Contents

CHAPTER 1

Introduction

1.1. The objectives of this book

The purpose of this book is the same as that of an edition written 4 years ago — to present information about energy balance in man which would be useful to the wide range of professions concerned with human obesity: physicians, dietitians, biochemists, physiologists, psychologists, physiotherapists and others. In that edition the introductory chapter ran to 38 pages to persuade all these people to think in terms of energy balance, and not to suppose that there was "a cause" of obesity, like overeating, inactivity, or some genetic disposition.

The situation has now changed. In the last 4 years there have been several major international congresses on obesity, energy balance, hunger and appetite, at which scientists from many disciplines have become much more familiar with the extraordinary variety of influences which may dispose to a positive energy balance, and hence obesity. Some of these hardly apply to the laboratory rat which was for so long a favourite model for the study of energy balance and its regulation. A long introduction is not necessary, but the recent explosion of literature in this field has made it very difficult to provide a concise and balanced review. Out of the about 500 references, carefully chosen 4 years ago, only 40% have survived the revision, and another 300 new ones have been added. No attempt has been made to be comprehensive in this bibliography: the publications cited are those which seemed to me to provide the best data relevant to the subject under discussion, but many good papers have been omitted in the interests of brevity. Most of the bibliography was published in the last 4 years, but some of the classics are irreplaceable and unsurpassed by anything published in the following half-century.

1.2. Lessons from the previous edition

I was surprised and very pleased by the way in which the first edition of this book was received. It is, of course, gratifying if reviewers comment favourably or provide constructive criticism, but better still to have received advice from all sorts of readers about the parts they found obscure, ambiguous, or simply wrong. I have tried to apply this criticism to improve the present version, and hope that readers will let me know which aspects they now find least satisfactory. Among the suggestions there were some that were mutually contradictory, but on some points there was agreement: first, there should be summaries at the end of each chapter; second, advice on the management of obese patients should be more specific; third, the book could be more concise.

Some readers tried, with varying degrees of directness, to discover the nature of my training and experience, or commercial associations. I am a general physician with an interest in obesity, employed solely by the Medical Research Council, and with no financial interest whatever in any food or pharmaceutical firm or slimming organisation of any kind. I have first and second hand experience (that is, I have both been the subject and the user) of all the methods for measuring energy intake and output mentioned in Chapter 3, and I have practical experience of giving and taking fat biopsies and trying all the methods of treatment on obese patients which are mentioned in Chapter 7 except chorionic gonadotrophin, jejunoileal bypass and stereotactic neurosurgery.

1.3. Recent advances in the field of energy balance and obesity

The major reorganisation of this text arises from the rapid advances which have been made in the last few years, both with techniques and interpretation.

Techniques for studying the control of food intake in man have become much more sophisticated, and the theoretical basis of this discipline has been revolutionised by the overthrow of the "dual centre" theory of a hunger and a satiety centre in the hypothalamus.

Conceptual models of food intake regulation in laboratory animals are complex, but it is generally recognised that in man the "big head problem" (see Section 4.4.1) introduces both metabolic and cognitive factors which no animal model can include.

Measurement of energy expenditure in man is now possible by direct calorimetry, an art forgotten by human physiologists for some 70 years. The classical studies of Atwater, Benedict and Boothby are now applicable to patients, and modern electronic techniques make them quite convenient both for the patient and the investigator. Direct calorimetry provides a very accurate reference standard against which the new indirect techniques, applicable to people going about their normal work, can be checked.

In the measurement of body composition the fallibility of traditional methods for estimating lean body mass has been established: particularly in very obese patients the ratio of water and potassium to other lean body components is not constant. However, very precise measurement of total body water by isotope mass spectrometry is now possible, and it may be feasible to measure density in a manner acceptable to patients. It is clearly established that rapid weight loss is not necessarily a characteristic of a good treatment for obesity, and that the influence of exercise on energy balance can only be assessed with the newer accurate measures of body composition, and not simply from weight change.

Recent work on the cellularity and metabolic activity of adipose tissue shows that "total fat cell number" is very difficult to determine in man, since the cells detected by current techniques do not include all potential fat cells. Generalisations about the association between early onset and hypercellular obesity have to be revised in the light of convincing evidence that hypercellularity is associated with severe obesity, not necessarily early onset obesity, although often the two categories apply to the same patient. There is no clear evidence to show if patients currently classified as "hypercellular" actually have more fat cells, or just have more of their fat cells storing fat.

In the treatment of obesity fashions come and go, but no single line of treatment has emerged as being generally effective. Progress in this field lies mostly in an increasing realisation that since the causes of obesity are so diverse there can be no panacaea, but rational investigation can indicate which treatments are likely to suit a given patient. Many forms of "protein sparing modified fast" are being advocated: there is remarkably little good evidence that any of them are superior in the long run to conventional reducing diets. The wave of enthusiasm for jejunoileal bypass as a treatment for severe obesity seems to have passed its peak: long-term complications are increasingly reported, and it is established that this operation has its effect by causing the patient to eat less. This end result can be achieved by less dangerous surgical procedures than those causing malabsorption, but it is not yet established if jaw wiring and gastric bypass is a satisfactory solution to the problem of grossly obese patients who are unable to reduce their food intake enough without some surgical assistance.

Negligible progress has been made in the prevention of obesity, since it has not proved possible to identify critical periods of development, or groups of individuals, where preventive measures would be particularly effective. The relationship of obesity to heart disease is now clearer: in middle-aged men without other risk factors the effect of overweight is small, but the association of overweight with excess mortality and morbidity in young people is well established, although the mechanism is still not clear.

CHAPTER 2

Definitions and usage

The purpose of this chapter is to list, for convenient reference, the manner in which terms and conventions have been used in this book. No special merit is claimed for these definitions over alternative definitions: they are chosen for clarity and convenience for the purpose of the argument here presented. Many of the definitions are not original, but their origins are not given unless the meaning of the term is usefully amplified in the original publication.

In situations where quotation is made from another author, who uses terms in a different sense, the difference in meaning is stated in the text at that point.

2.1. Units for the measurement of energy: kilogramme calorie (kcal) and joule (J)

In most of the literature which has been reviewed in this book energy has been measured in kilogramme calories, variously abbreviated kcal, Cal, or cal. The Royal Society Conference of Editors (1968) recommended that the system of units known as SI should be adopted in all scientific and technical journals, and consequently publications are using SI units for most purposes and generally this causes no practical problems. The conversion from litre to dm^3, for example, is of only academic interest to most nutritionists, since the difference in the two units is only 27 parts per million, and nutritional measurements are not of this order of accuracy. In the case of measurements of energy the problem is more difficult, since the SI equivalent of the calorie is the joule. The precise conversion factor is 4.183 J = 1 calorie.

The practice which has been adopted in this book is to quote val-

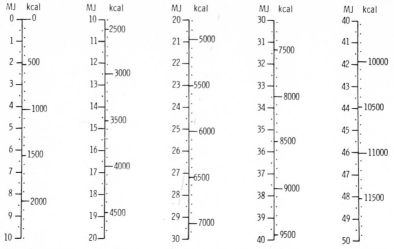

Fig. 2.1. Scale to facilitate conversion of energy units between megajoules (MJ) and kilocalories (kcal).

ues in kcal where they were originally so published, and to provide (in parentheses) the equivalent in joules where this seems appropriate.

The precise conversion factor has not been used, but a rounded conversion factor appropriate to the accuracy of the measurement discussed. It is hoped that this compromise solution will be satisfactory during the period of transition between the two systems of measurement. A scale is given in Fig. 2.1 to facilitate conversion between megajoules and kilocalories.

2.2. Body composition and obesity

Obesity is a condition caused by an excessive amount of adipose tissue. The advantages and limitations of this definition are discussed in Chapter 7.1.

2.2.1. Fat and adipose tissue

Fat consists of glyceryl esters of fatty acids. There are two advantages in defining obesity as "excessive accumulation of body fat" as

Mayer and others have done (Mayer, 1970). The first is that people do not gain and lose fat alone as they become more or less obese, they gain and lose mostly tissue from beneath the skin, of which the chemical composition is shown in Table 7.1. Roughly 80% of the weight of this adipose tissue is fat, about 2% is protein and the remainder water. In the normal subject, in whom the mass of adipose tissue is fairly constant, it does not matter much if no distinction is made between fat and adipose tissue, but in the obese subject who loses, say, 50 kg of adipose tissue it causes a considerable error if this weight loss is calculated as fat, both in terms of the change in energy stores and also the composition of the lean body mass.

The second difficulty with the definition of obesity in terms of fat is that total body fat is very difficult to measure (see 6.2.2), and the skinfold calipers recommended by Mayer really measure subcutaneous adipose tissue. It is therefore convenient to use the term "fat" when the chemical substance is meant, and "adipose tissue" for the less well defined mixture of fat, water and protein.

2.2.2. Water and fluid retention

Water, like fat, is a definite chemical compound. It can be measured in tissue samples by desiccation, and in living human subjects by tracer dilution techniques (see 6.2.2). If, in a normal human subject, total body water is increased or decreased there is a corresponding change in solute, so that the osmolarity of the tissues is little changed.

The term "fluid retention" is not used in this book. It has been used by others to explain changes in body weight not accompanied by significant changes in energy balance, and the impression is created that changes of a few kilogrammes may occur in a quite arbitrary manner. This is untrue. In a normal subject, who is given an oral load of 1000 ml of water, a diuresis starts within 15–30 min, and within 3 h the excess water has been cleared. True "fluid retention" may, of course, occur in people with heart failure or renal disease. To a large extent the phenomenon of "fluid retention" in normal subjects can be explained by changes in the glycogen–water pool (see 2.2.4).

2.2.3. Fat-free body and lean body mass

The fat-free body is the sum of all the tissues of the body minus the total body fat. This can be measured in living subjects if fat is estimated either by fat-soluble gas techniques (6.2.1) or by density (6.3.2). The composition of the fat-free bodies of 6 adult cadavers is shown in Table 6.1.

Lean body mass is the sum of all the tissues of the body minus the adipose tissue. The difference between fat and adipose tissue was explained in 2.2.1. The difference between lean body mass and fat-free body is that, by definition, lean body mass remains constant in composition (but not necessarily in quantity) with increasing and decreasing obesity, whereas the composition of the fat-free body clearly changes. This is important, since methods of estimating lean body mass, either by density or by whole body potassium content, depend on an assumed constant composition.

2.2.4. The glycogen—water pool

The work of Olsson and Saltin (1970) has shown that by manipulating diet and exercise it is possible to alter the size of the muscle glycogen store over a range of about 500 g. This was confirmed by analysis of needle biopsies of muscle. They also showed that each gramme of glycogen bound 3—4 g water. The glycogen—water pool is the total mass of this glycogen—water mixture in the body.

It is not possible to measure the size of this pool directly, but its behaviour during states of energy imbalance can be inferred indirectly. The postulated magnitude of the pool corresponds well with the fast component of weight loss during starvation (see 7.2.1), and with the change in body weight with isocaloric substitution of carbohydrate in a reducing diet.

Direct evidence that the glycogen—water pool acts as a labile energy store in a subject who is approximately in energy balance may be obtained by means of an experiment such as that illustrated in Fig. 2.2. During the 10 days of this experiment there were minor energy imbalances of a few hundred kcal at the beginning and end of the *ad libitum* feeding periods. Since the subject was weighed twice daily under standard conditions it is possible to relate the weight change during each of the 20 half-day periods to the change in energy balance during these half-day periods. If the weight change is at the expense of a glycogen—water pool there should be a significant relationship between weight change and energy imbalance, whereas if weight change is related to "fluid retention" unrelated to energy stores no such relationship would be expected.

The result of plotting weight change against energy imbalance for each half-day period is shown in Fig. 2.2. The regression line has a slope of 1.07, indicating that there was a change in weight of approximately 1 g for every 1 kcal (4.2 kJ) energy imbalance. The correlation is significant ($r = 0.91$; $P < 0.001$). This demonstrates that there is some labile energy store with a value of 1 kcal/g which is used to cover small changes in energy balance. In view of the other evidence presented above, the obvious candidate for this energy store is the glycogen—water pool, which has all the correct characteristics to act in this way.

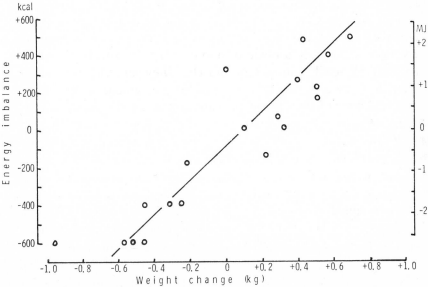

Fig. 2.2. Relationship of weight change to small degrees of energy imbalance in a normal subject. The regression line has a slope indicating a change in weight of approximately 1 g/kcal energy imbalance: this corresponds to a glycogen—water mixture with 1 g of glycogen binding 3 g of water.

2.3. Energy intake and expenditure

"Energy intake" normally means the metabolisable energy in the food. When the diet contains protein and unavailable carbohydrate (such as cellulose) the total heat of combustion of the food is greater than the metabolisable energy, the yield of energy from protein by total combustion in a bomb calorimeter to carbon dioxide and water is greater than that by oxidation in the body to urea. Cellulose in the diet will likewise give a value of 4 kcal/g (17 kJ) on combustion in the bomb calorimeter, but since this material cannot be digested in the human gut this energy is not available for metabolic purposes. Strictly speaking "energy intake" should mean energy absorbed from the food, but this is difficult to measure. In normal subjects the energy content of the faeces is about 3–8% of energy intake, but not all of this is material which has passed through the gut unabsorbed: some has been secreted into the gut. Often energy intake is calculated by reference to food tables in which digestibility had already been taken into account in calculating the energy value of the food.

"Energy expenditure" is the total heat output of the subject, including the equivalent heat of water vaporised. In practice it is rarely measured directly, but it is estimated by various methods which are discussed in Chapter 3.

2.3.1. Energy balance

If the energy intake of a subject equals his energy output (or expenditure) then he is in energy balance, and energy stores remain constant. If intake exceeds output he is in positive balance, and if output exceeds intake he is in negative balance.

The concept of a subject in energy balance is a theoretical abstraction, since in any subject the state of balance varies from minute to minute. For practical purposes we may take agreement between measured intake and output of energy within 50 kcal (210 kJ) per day as representing energy balance, owing to the limited accuracy with which intake and output can be measured. However, if a person maintains a constant body weight over a period of 10 years this represents a mean error of energy balance of less than 2 kcal (8 kJ) per day.

2.3.2. Appetite, hunger and satiety

The distinction between hunger and appetite made by Yudkin (1963) is that hunger is a sensation which makes one want to eat; appetite is a sensation which makes one want to eat a particular food. This seems a sensible use of words, but one which is often not followed. For example anorectic drugs are usually said to control appetite, but in fact they act on hunger. Hypothalamic lesions in rats affect hunger: it is usually not known if they affect appetite, since it is impossible to distinguish between hunger and appetite if only one food is offered.

Satiety is impossible to define with any precision. It is a sensation intermediate between the relief of hunger and the nausea which ultimately limits overeating.

The "eating behaviour" described by psychologists in subjects who are bored, apprehensive or depressed seems to be unconnected with any of the sensations discussed above. Obese patients may report that they have overeaten, but at the same time deny that they had been hungry. It appears that a word is missing from the vocabulary available to describe eating behaviour.

2.4. Control and regulation

The use of these words is based on that of Brobeck (1965). A quantity which is regulated is maintained at a constant value ("kept regular"), and to achieve this regulation other rates of working must be controlled or adjusted. Thus a thermostat controls the output of a heating device in order to regulate the temperature of a room.

2.5. Statistical methods and conventions

A difference is described as "not significant" if statistical tests indicate that such a difference might have arisen by chance more than once in 20 times.

Throughout this book a standard notation will be used: n for the number of subjects, S.D. for standard deviation, and P for test of statistical probability.

In ordinary English the terms "accuracy" and "precision" are often used interchangeably. Strictly the accuracy of a measurement depends on how closely the answer resembles the true answer, and precision relates to the reproducibility with which a measurement can be made. These are not necessarily the same, as the following example illustrates.

Suppose a group of people are asked to guess the weight of a man who weighs 70.00 kg. Their estimates may range from 65 kg to 75 kg, and the mean of these estimates might be 70 kg. If the same observers are then asked to weigh the man on a balance which has been badly calibrated they will produce a new set of estimates which might range from 68.9 to 69.1 kg, so this set of weighings would be more precise, but less accurate, than the original set of guesses.

If we attempt to assess the accuracy of a method for measuring (for example) the total body fat in a living man the task is very difficult. If the total fat in the man was known there would be no need to devise a method for estimating it. If it is not known the accuracy can only be inferred by the precision of the measurement (which may be misleading, as shown above), or by the extent to which the answer resembles that obtained by any alternative methods which may be available.

The correlation coefficient, conventionally represented "r", indicates how closely two variables are linked. If they are perfectly correlated, like the number of postage stamps bought in a year, and the number sold in the same year, $r = 1.0$. If the printing of stamps is efficiently organised there will also be a high correlation (say $r = 0.95$) between the number printed and the number sold. In the biological sciences it can be very difficult to interpret correctly moderately strong correlations; for example in a group of 13 grossly obese women the correlation between oxygen uptake and body weight was 0.57, between oxygen uptake and lean body mass 0.55, and between oxygen uptake and total fat 0.62. Therefore it was concluded (see p. 85) that fat is the body component which most closely relates to oxygen uptake. However this conclusion depends entirely on the data from the most extremely obese patient in the group. If she is omitted and correlation coefficients for oxygen uptake are calculated for the remaining 12 patients they are 0.81, 0.77 and 0.71 for body weight, lean body mass and total fat respectively, and so the original conclusion is reversed by the omission of a single patient. It is therefore necessary to be very careful when drawing conclusions from correlation coefficients of about 0.6 based on fairly small numbers of observations.

2.6. Statistical versus biological significance: common mistakes

Statistical techniques help biologists to judge if the results they obtain are likely to have arisen by chance, but there are three ways in which they are commonly misused.

2.6.1. The "constancy" fallacy

If an investigator fails to show that a measurement changes significantly this does not entitle him to claim that he has shown that it is "constant". For example with weight loss the apparent number of fat cells in obese patients sometimes increases and sometimes decreases (Björntorp et al., 1975), so on average the change is not significantly different from zero. This result may be interpreted to mean that these changes in different directions really occur in different people, or alternatively that the error of the measurement is such that the observed changes may not be real, but it cannot be taken to mean that cell number has been shown to be constant.

2.6.2. The "prediction" fallacy

Many workers measure several variables in a group of people, have a multiple regression analysis done on a computer, and find to their delight that they have found a means of "predicting" some value (like total body fat) from their measurements with greater accuracy than by any previously published equation. They will henceforth maintain that the inclusion of a particular circumference or skinfold is the secret of the superiority of their equation. In fact, their equation works well for their series because it was derived from that series. To test its predictive power it should now be used on a new

14

TABLE 2.1

AN EXERCISE IN THE PREDICTION OF NON-EXISTENT RELATIONSHIPS

	Series 1		Series 2	
	x	y	x	y
	20	17	74	49
	42	28	04	49
	23	17	03	04
	59	66	10	33
	38	61	53	70
	02	10	11	54
	86	10	48	63
	51	55	94	60
	92	52	94	49
	44	25	57	38
Correlation (*r*)	0.377		0.477	
Slope (b)	0.295		0.276	
Intercept (a)	20.6		35.8	

series of subjects, and it may well turn out that the extra circumference or skinfold has no predictive power at all.

The ease with which it is possible to derive "prediction equations" from data which are totally non-significant is shown in Table 2.1.

If the values in the columns headed x and y had been measurements, and an investigator wished to produce a formula by which, from a knowledge of x the value of y could be "predicted", the best formula for the data in series 1 would be y = 20.6 + 0.295x, and in series 2 a still better prediction could be obtained from the formula y = 35.8 + 0.276x.

In fact the values in Table 2.1 are the first two lines of figures from the table of random sampling numbers, from p. 16 of the Cambridge Elementary Statistical Tables, edited by Lindley and Miller (1964), and are as non-significant as it is possible for numbers to be. The sceptical reader can repeat the exercise from any set of random numbers and confirm for himself two facts which it is useful to remember: (1) it is always possible to find a "best fit" line to any data, however meaningless they may be, and (2) "prediction formulae" work best when used on the data from which they were derived.

2.6.3. The "double six" fallacy

The chance that a player on his first throw of a pair of dice will get a double six is about 0.03, so an observer who sees this happen might believe that he had "statistically significant" evidence that the dice were loaded, but, as Peto and Doll (1977) observe, "it would clearly be foolish to believe this on all occasions." The reference cited is part of an interesting correspondence in which a most distinguished statistician points out that probability values indicate probability, and there is nothing disreputable about using a certain amount of common sense in their interpretation.

CHAPTER 3

Methods for measuring energy intake and output: their use and misuse

3.1. Measurement of energy intake

It is very difficult to make an accurate measurement of what people normally eat. If patients are confined in a metabolic ward with security arrangements more appropriate to a prison (Garrow et al., 1978), what they eat can be measured accurately but is probably not normal. If dietary survey techniques are used to assess habitual diet (Marr, 1971) the measured intake is normal but not very accurate. There is no escape from this dilemma. Since in the study of energy balance accuracy is essential, we will start with techniques which provide accurate measurements at the expense of acceptability and progress towards methods of measuring intake which are more spontaneous but less accurate.

3.1.1. Dispensed liquid diets

To calculate energy intake from the diet it is necessary to multiply the quantity of each item of food consumed by the concentration of energy in each item, and to sum the contribution of all the components of the diet. Obviously if the diet consists solely of one item of food, both analysis and calculation are greatly simplified. Furthermore if the diet consists of a homogeneous liquid, such as milk, it is very easy to take a representative sample for analysis. Thus the dispensed, liquid diet is ideal for the most accurate measurement of intake, and the food intake of infants has been measured with great precision in the metabolic ward (Chan and Waterlow, 1966) or even in children living at home (Fomon et al., 1971). Individually packed baby feeds are now commercially available, so it is practicable to provide the mother with a supply of bottles containing a known amount of a liquid food of known composition. If the bottle is collected and reweighed after the baby has been fed, it is possible to calculate the energy intake with a high degree of accuracy, making the sole assumption that everything which has left the bottle has entered the baby. This assumption will be incorrect in the case of a baby who regurgitates food, but, compared with most other methods, the accuracy of this technique is very high.

Unfortunately dispensed liquid diets are less satisfactory for studies on adults. The theoretical advantages remain, but in practice it may be very difficult to obtain meaningful results. For example, Campbell et al. (1971) used a food-dispensing apparatus to study the ability of obese and lean subjects to adjust their intake, when the caloric density of the liquid diet was changed. The lean subjects were 5 healthy male students, and the obese subjects were 2 adolescent boys and 4 women aged 25–30 years. In all the subjects, when the diet was changed from a hospital diet of conventional food to liquid formula intake by machine, the body weight dropped, but thereafter the lean subjects maintained weight fairly well by making appropriate adjustments when the nutritive density was varied. On the other hand, the obese subjects (according to the authors' own abstract) "seem incapable of such regulation". One obese subject, R.M., is discussed in detail, and was said to show a "paradoxical drop in volume intake when the nutritive density of the formula was decreased." Inspection of the data suggests that subject R.M., a 30-year-old lady who weighed 143 kg, just was not prepared to feed herself from the machine. She was studied for 5 periods, the first 4 lasted 10 days each, and the fifth 13 days. The average volume of diet which she took from the machine decreased steadily throughout the experiment, from 441 ml/day in the first period to 189 ml/day in the fifth. At no stage did she obtain more than 660 kcal (2.8 MJ) per day from the machine. Clearly, therefore, her feeding behaviour during the 53 days of this study cannot have resembled that of the previous 30 years, or she would not have weighed 143 kg.

3.1.2. Mixed diets composed of selected items

Liquid dispensed diets are monotonous and hence, as shown in the example quoted above, unsuitable for the study of normal eating behaviour. A more attractive and better tolerated diet can be devised by careful selection of foods to provide a uniformity, and hence suitability for analysis, comparable to that of liquid diets. In the meticulous study by Southgate and Durnin (1970) groups of volunteers ate 3 different experimental diets for metabolic balance periods of 7 days each, with a run-in period of 2–3 days on the diet before collections began. The purpose of the investigation was to re-assess the conversion factors which are used to calculate the energy value of the diet from its protein, fat and carbohydrate content. Every effort was therefore made to ensure that the diet consumed was identical to that which was taken for analysis: fat was trimmed from meat, and frying was not used as a means of cooking. All meals were closely supervised, and two or more observers lived with the subjects in their hostel or hall of residence. The conclusion of the investigation was that the calorie conversion factors used in the food tables of McCance and Widdowson (1960) are satisfactory, since the mean difference between the energy value of the diets calculated using these factors, and that found by direct bomb calorimetry of the diet, was only 1.87%. It is interesting, however, to note that with some diets, in some groups of subjects, there is a difference of 4% in the mean value by the two methods. If we assume direct bomb calorimetry to be the standard by which all other methods of estimating energy intake should be judged, this suggests that even the most carefully selected diet may have a calculated energy content significantly different from the true value. If there is no systematic error in the method of calculation (and the data suggest that there is not), and if the mean value for 12 subjects eating a diet for 7 days is sometimes 4% wrong, statistical considerations suggest that for some of those subjects, at some time, the calculated value would be 10% out.

Foods with a high fibre content are also unsuitable for accurate calorimetry. In the bomb calorimeter the complex carbohydrates in some vegetable foods will burn to give a total energy value, but in the human digestive tract the hemicelluloses, for example, are not digested by intestinal enzymes and are only slightly broken down by normal gut microorganisms. Indeed the presence of a large amount of fibre actually reduces the amount of available energy by hastening the passage of food through the gut and diminishing the absorption of protein and fat (Southgate and Durnin, 1970). In the 1960 edition of "The Composition of Foods", Dr. Widdowson reviews the possible methods of calculating caloric values, and explains why they have expressed "available carbohydrate" as monosaccharides, and used the factor 3.75 to convert to calories. A table on page 177 shows that 3 different methods of calculating calorie conversion yield results which agree within 2% or so. The alternative to the method of estimating separately, and then summing, the caloric contribution of glucose, fructose, sucrose, dextrins and starch (which is the method used in McCance and Widdowson's food tables) is to estimate "fibre" directly. This involves successive extractions with petroleum spirit, boiling dilute sulphuric acid, boiling dilute sodium hydroxide solution, dilute hydrochloric acid, alcohol and finally ether. Even after all this effort "the recovery of cellulose using the specified procedure seldom exceeds four-fifths of that actually present ..." (Pearson, 1970).

Some clinicians have a misplaced faith in the reliability of duplicate diet analysis. Even if they are fortunate in having a laboratory which will perform a precise analysis on the "duplicate diet" (that is, a collection of the same weight and type of food as that given to the patient), there are two sources of error which are difficult to avoid. The first is the inhomogeneity of many foods; for example the energy value of raw bacon varies from 355 to 612 kcal (0.15–0.26 MJ) per 100 g according to the fat content of the particular cut used. The food tables give a value of 7 kcal (0.03 MJ) per 100 g for raw mushrooms, and 217 kcal (0.91 MJ) for mushrooms fried in dripping, so obviously it matters very much how they are cooked, and if the sample transferred to the duplicate diet container is exactly similar to that which the patient eats. The second cause of error is plate waste, which may be difficult to calculate. The energy content of a salad dressed with oil may be calculated, but the energy consumed depends on how much oil is left on the plate.

An ingenious development in using mixed diets has been suggested by Silverstone (1978). He uses a snack vending machine to provide experimental diets for studies on food intake, and thus avoids many of the disadvantages of both liquid dispensed diets and freely chosen diets, while preserving most of the advantages. The vending machine is loaded with items such as sandwiches, portions of fruit, pieces of chocolate and similar items, each individually wrapped in plastic film. The diet is therefore much more varied and interesting than a liquid diet, but items can be chosen which are homogeneous and easy to analyse, and there is no problem with plate waste.

Thus it is difficult to say how accurately one can measure the energy content of a mixed diet which has been prepared in a diet kitchen to meet the food preferences of the subject. If the subject insists on deriving the majority of his energy from food such as bacon, fried mushrooms, fruit in syrup, bran and salad dressed with oil then it is unlikely that the estimate will be better than 5% in error, while with a subject who is satisfied with foods such as white bread, butter and jelly, eggs and milk, it is possible, with care, to approach the accuracy of liquid diets.

3.1.3. Weighed freely chosen diets

This is the method used by Widdowson (1936) in her classical study of the daily food intake of 63 middle-class men. Each subject was provided with a spring balance weighing by 0.25 oz. up to 1 lb, a plate on which to weigh the food, and a form on which to enter the results. Every item of food eaten during 1 week was weighed, and the calorie content was calculated from food tables. It is not possible to provide an exact figure for the intrinsic errors in this method, because it will obviously depend on how conscientious the subjects were in their weighing and recording, and the extent to which this unfamiliar process altered their normal eating habits. In the case of pies, stews, cakes and puddings the food table values are based on assumed recipes, so the results will be wrong to the extent that the recipes used by the subjects differed from that used by the compilers of food tables. One may reasonably suppose, however, that given intelligent and cooperative subjects the error of this method should not be more than 5–10%.

It can be argued that the weighed inventory method is *only* suitable for intelligent and cooperative subjects, and that selection of subjects may introduce significant bias. Marr (1971) reviews 7 surveys which used this method, and shows that the yield of valid returns varied from about one-third to two-thirds of the population surveyed. Thomson (1958) showed that the subjects failing to make returns were more likely to be younger, less intelligent and of lower social class than the average for the group. Another limitation of the weighed inventory method is that it is unsuitable for those who often eat away from home. To some extent the demands on the subject can be reduced by asking them to record their intake in "standard household measures" such as cupfuls or spoonfuls. Obviously an infinite gradation is possible, from "50 g potato" through "two small potatoes" to "not much potato", and one can only make the general comment that accuracy is attainable only at the expense of subject cooperation, and vice versa.

3.1.4. Dietary records or diaries

The principal merit of this technique is that it is applicable to unsophisticated subjects, as for example the Trinidadian women studied by McCarthy (1966). The plan was to ask the subjects, some obese and some not obese, to keep a 7-day food diary in which they recorded, in household measures, what they ate. They were interviewed by the same nutritionist twice, approximately one week apart, and cross-checks, such as 24 h recalls and spot checks on the frequency of consumption of certain foods, were made. Of the 184 initial appointments which were made, 125 were kept. Completed diaries and second interviews were obtained from 102 subjects, but 13 of these were later disqualified, so the final yield was about a third of the initial sample. The calorie intake of 26 control subjects was calculated to be 1978 (S.D. 479) kcal/day, and of 63 obese subjects 1884 (S.D. 534) kcal/day: the difference is not statistically significant. Estimates of physical activity, obtained by recall methods, also failed to distinguish between the two groups. It is obvious that, in this survey, the methods used were totally inadequate to detect the cause of energy imbalance in the obese women. What is less obvious is what practicable alternative one might suggest. This topic is discussed further in 3.3.

There are several papers in which the inadequacy of the data cannot be excused by lack of sophistication among the subjects surveyed. In my experience the prize for sheer optimism in the interpretation of useless data should go to Lincoln (1972). He too was concerned with the relative contribution of overeating and inactivity to the causation of obesity, so he inquired, by postal questionnaire, about the food intake (for one 24-h period) and physical activity of 867 men. Predictably, he failed to find the cause of obesity, but noted, as others have done, that fat people tend to say that they have eaten less than thin people do.

3.1.5. Retrospective estimate by recall or interview

The limitations of a technique based simply on asking the subject what he has recently eaten are obvious. The longer the period which he tries to remember the less accurate is his recollection likely to be. Dietary recall of the previous 24 h is therefore sometimes used as a check on other methods, but it is hardly worth considering as a method in itself.

However, the method of Burke (1947) is intended to determine the dietary pattern of the subject over several months or years. The method is extensively used in clinical practice and is potentially very valuable, since, if the reconstruction of dietary pattern is accurate, it is clearly a "habitual" food intake: unlike any prospective method, the dietary history method cannot be accused of influencing the thing which it seeks to measure. The problem, of course, is to show that the estimate is an accurate one, and many attempts at validation have been made.

Reed and Burke (1954) used the dietary history method to calculate the protein and energy intake of children aged 1–6 years. They compared the results with the growth rate of the children and concluded that their estimate of protein intake was usually correct within 10 g. This is roughly equivalent to saying that the standard deviation of the estimate from the true value for protein intake would be 10%. As Mayer (1952) has commented, "current methods of dietary intake studies show a much greater imprecision regarding calories than regarding other nutrients, such as protein", so this would indicate a greater than 10% standard deviation for calories by the Burke interview method. Furthermore, as Reed and Burke (1954) themselves say, the method requires a cooperative and intelligent informant, a trained interviewer, and a standard procedure. Many people who say they use the Burke method do not in fact follow the original design. This was in 3 parts: first the interviewer established the dietary pattern by a series of questions about what was actually eaten at each meal in the recent past, and whether this was typical or not of that meal in general, and the extent to which the meal pattern was altered when the subject was away from home, or at weekends; next came a series of cross-checks and special questions to confirm or refute impressions about the dietary pattern, for example the total amount of various foods purchased weekly; finally the subject recorded his actual intake for 3 days. The last step is now commonly omitted. The interview normally takes about an hour, and if it is found that day-to-day variations are too great "it may be impossible to determine average daily food intake" (Reed and Burke, 1954).

Beaudoin and Mayer (1953) compared the calorie intake of obese and non-obese women calculated from 1-day and 3-day food records, or from dietary interview. They concluded that while the 3 methods gave similar results for women of average weight, for obese women "individual food recording methods gave grossly inadequate mean calorie intakes. The research dietary history yielded results in agreement with physiologic considerations", that is, higher intakes. From a careful reading of the text it is doubtful if this conclusion is justified by the data. It is clear that the 3 methods were applied to different obese women. Thus the average for 1-day food records on 59 obese women was 1964 kcal/day, for 3-day food records from 12 obese women (not included in the first group) was 1591 kcal/day, and by research dietary history from either 33 or 53 obese women (text and tables give contradictory figures) the average intake was calculated to be 2829 kcal/day. It is not clear what this tells us about the accuracy of any of the methods.

Trulson (1954) compared the food intake of children assessed by either a 7-day weighed record, a research dietary interview, or 3 or more 24-h recalls. Mean values by the 3 methods were similar, and 7-day records and dietary history results agreed better than the 24-h recall method. She concluded that the dietary interview was the method of choice, and that the differences between the methods were inconsistent for different foods. Van den Berg and Mayer (1954) tested the 1-day recorded intake and research dietary interview on 35 obese pregnant women, who were given a record sheet and instructed to enter the food they ate during any one day of the week. The majority chose weekdays, and only 4, Saturday or Sunday. The mean intake from these records was 1763 (S.D. 514) kcal/day. The next week a research dietary interview was done by an experienced interviewer who had no knowledge of the result of the 1-day record. The mean value from the interview was 2354 (S.D. 600) kcal/day. The difference is significant at the 1% level. In particular the dietary history elicited information about between meal snacks which had not appeared on the recorded intake, and the estimate of the quantities of foods, particularly carbohydrate ones, was greater by interview than by record. The authors conclude, therefore, that the fact that intake is being recorded significantly reduces the amount that is eaten.

3.1.6. The obese dieter

So far we have considered ways in which it is possible to measure the food intake of normal subjects who are eating, if not entirely freely, at least so as to satisfy their hunger. Special problems arise when one tries to find out if an obese patient, who has been prescribed a reducing diet, is in fact keeping to the diet. Some clinicians are so cynical as to say that this problem is in practice easy to solve: if the patient is losing weight he (or more commonly she) is keeping to the diet, and if weight is not being lost this is because the patient is "cheating". This approach is highly satisfactory from the viewpoint of the clinician, since the basic tenet is that the doctor's remedy is always effective if conscientiously applied. It follows with inexorable logic that any failure must therefore be a failure on the part of the patient, who has only him- (or her-)self to blame.

From the viewpoint of the patient the situation is less satisfactory. There are situations, which are discussed more fully in Chapter 7, in which an obese person may have a mean calorie intake of 1000 kcal (4.2 MJ) per day but be losing less than 1 kg/week. Usually this will be a middle aged woman who has lost perhaps 10 or 20 kg with a view to becoming eligible for some orthopaedic operation, but who is told by the surgeon that she must lose another 10 or 20 kg before he is willing to operate. If she has found that her rate of weight loss is by now very slow, even with strict adherence to the diet, her outlook is bleak; and if, when she consults her dietary advisor, she is told that her failure to lose weight must be proof of "cheating" on the diet, this is unlikely to raise her spirits. Indeed these people become understandably depressed and easy prey for charlatans with magic slimming cures. The mechanism by which calorie requirements may become unusually low is discussed elsewhere (see 5.1.4). How, then, can one distinguish between an obese patient who is not losing weight, is very sorry for herself, and *is* keeping to a low energy diet, and another patient who is equally statically obese, equally melancholy, but who is *not* keeping to the diet? In short, can one diagnose cheating?

It is (I believe) always possible to diagnose cheating, although in some cases it can be very difficult. A skillful and experienced dietitian will form a much more accurate estimate of a patient's true energy intake than a physician unversed in this art. However, the chronic cheater also becomes skillful and experienced in handling her case in the dietetic interview, and after many years of dietetic interrogation, and having read innumerable diet sheets, the patient becomes at least as familiar with the "correct" answers as the dietitian herself. It is sometimes said that if the patient cheats and does not confess that this is so, it is a waste of time to attempt further treatment. There is great force in this argument. Most doctors will know of massively obese patients who are constantly seeking sympathy for their plight, but who seem unwilling to make the slightest effort on their own behalf. However, dietary histories in severely obese patients are seldom as simple as they seem. The fact that the patient is obese, and has come for advice, indicates that the mechanism of energy balance is unusual in this person. Such a person is subject to all sorts of social pressures which the lean person does not experience, and it is not uncommon for the obese patient to have quite extraordinary ideas about what would usually be regarded as a "normal" diet. These aberrations may be either overestimates or underestimates. Thus one patient may be entirely convinced that she has "eaten practically nothing all week" when her intake has averaged 2000 kcal (8.4 MJ) per day, while another may confess to having "gone wild" on the occasion of some family gathering, when in fact the total departure from the prescribed diet amounted to about 400 kcal (1.7 MJ) on one occasion.

If any seriously obese patient (say, one who is disabled by obesity, or who, although at present asymptomatic, is 20 or more kg over-weight) is unable to lose at least 6 kg in 3 months, then it is useful to discover the reason for failure. In order to distinguish between the refractory obese with abnormally low requirements, and those who persistently cheat on the diet, it may well be necessary to employ the tests of energy expenditure described in Chapter 5. Even when they are admitted to a metabolic ward for investigation some patients will try to produce false results to confuse the diagnosis. The motives behind these actions are discussed elsewhere (see Chapter 7). The obese dieter is given a special section in this discussion on the errors inherent in various methods of measuring food intake because they present a special problem, and it is necessary to realise that, delibe-rately or otherwise, some of these patients may succeed in misleading even the most competent investigators.

3.2. Methods for measuring energy expenditure

The same comments which were made in 3.1 about the "uncer-tainty principle" in the measurement of energy intake apply with equal force to the measurement of energy expenditure. The highest accuracy is only to be obtained at the cost of inconvenience, both to investigator and subject, which by present-day standards amounts to hardship. It is worth considering in some detail the experiments of the great pioneers in this field, which will illustrate this statement.

3.2.1. The direct calorimeter

"Every year I have the pleasure of describing Atwater's beautiful experiments to a new class of medical students. . . . it is possible to make measurements on a human subject over a period of several days with the precision customary in the physical sciences" (Passmore, 1967). It is possible indeed, but only with skill, vigilance and dedication.

The Atwater calorimeter was developed and perfected over a period of 12 years, and a description of the final instrument is given in great detail by Atwater and Benedict (1905). It was situated in a basement room in the Orange Judd Hall of the Wesleyan University, at Middletown, Conn.: a Holy Place to any student of energy balance in man. The calorimeter chamber was essentially a box 2.15 m long, 1.22 m wide and 1.93 m high, made from sheets of 24-gauge copper soldered together. The subject entered through an aperture 49 cm wide and 70 cm high, which was then sealed with a sheet of plate glass bedded in melted beeswax. The chamber was furnished with a table and a bed, both of which could be folded away when not in use, a chair, a telephone, and a bicycle ergometer. There was no source of light inside the chamber, but the aperture faced an outside window of the building.

Completely surrounding the copper chamber and separated from it by an air space of 7.6 cm was another box made of sheet zinc. Surrounding the zinc box were two further concentric coverings of wood, again with an air space of about 7 cm between them. To detect differences in temperature between the copper and zinc shells there were 304 pairs of thermocouples bridging the air gap at selected points over the entire surface of the chamber, and provision was made for heating or cooling the air outside the zinc shell to ensure that the two metal shells could be held at the same temperature at all times, whatever the change in heat production within the copper chamber. Thus escape of heat through the walls of the chamber was prevented.

In order to remove heat from the chamber as fast as it was produced by the subject, water was circulated through cooling pipes inside the chamber. The temperature of the ingoing and outgoing water was read from specially calibrated mercury thermometers to 0.01°C, and the flow rate of water was monitored by an ingenious system which weighed the outcoming water in pans which held about 10 kg water. As one pan became full the flow was switched to another, and the weight of the pan was determined to 2 g. When the subject was asleep at night 10 kg of water, entering at about 5°C and leaving at about 15°C, would suffice to keep the calorimeter at 20°C for 2 or 3 h. When the subject was hard at work 10 kg water might last only 7 min. Throughout the experiments, which lasted from 1 to 13 days, a team of observers kept records of the temperature of the various layers of the calorimeter wall, and of the cooling water, and of the air which was pumped through the calorimeter at 75 l/min, and that of the subject (by rectal thermometer) every 4 min. After each reading the flow rate of the cooling water, and the temperature of the air outside the zinc shell, was adjusted so as to maintain a constant temperature in the calorimeter chamber, and a zero temperature gradient across the walls. Each experimental day was divided into four 6-h periods, starting at 07.00 h. Thus at 07.00, 13.00, 19.00 and 01.00 h there was a stocktaking of the total amount of heat removed by the cooling water, and by the water vapour in the expired air. Carbon dioxide production was calculated by the change in weight of soda lime absorbers, the composition of the gas in the calorimeter was analysed, and the subject, his clothing and bedding were weighed to correct for changes in humidity.

If the experimental procedure was exacting, the calculations were no less laborious. Corrections had to be made for the thermal mass of the calorimeter walls (60 kcal/°C); for the thermal mass and temperature of all food entering, or excreta leaving, the calorimeter; for changes in atmospheric pressure (since with a volume of about 5000 litres a change of 1 mm Hg in barometric pressure represents a change of over 6 litres in effective gas volume); and many other minor factors. In the circumstances it is understandable that by 1905, after 12 years of development, these indefatigable workers had completed only 22 experiments on 5 human subjects. This section is concerned with direct calorimetry, so it is this aspect of the work which is here described, but simultaneously Atwater and Benedict were doing complete metabolic balance studies, including complete measurements of gas exchange.

The precision of the results was indeed awe-inspiring. There were two standard calibration checks for the calorimeter; the electrical check and the alcohol lamp check. A known amount of heat was generated inside the calorimeter by these means. For a known dissipation of heat from an electric fire 99.72% was recovered, and the recoveries of the products of combustion of a known amount of ethyl alcohol were for heat 99.8%, for carbon dioxide produced 100.1%, for water produced 100.6% and for oxygen consumed 101.0%.

With a human subject as the source of heat the results were less precise, but still magnificent by modern standards. Atwater and Benedict (1899) report the results of their first experiments on man. In each case the subject was Mr. E. Osterberg, a man of 31 years "in excellent health and accustomed, as laboratory janitor and chemical assistant, to moderate muscular labour". The first 4 experiments were primarily concerned with calibration or were "so vitiated by accident as not to be completed". The results of experiments 5–10 are shown in Table 3.1.

The authors comment on the unsatisfactory discrepancy between predicted and observed heat production in Experiment 5, an error of 4.1%. This they ascribe principally to the diet which was more varied than that of some of the later experiments. Mr. Osterberg's tolerance seems to have been as excellent as his health, because he ate the experimental diet for 8 days before entering the calorimeter, instead of the normal 4 days, as unexpected circumstances delayed the start

TABLE 3.1

SUMMARY OF ENERGY BALANCE IN MAN BY DIRECT CALORIMETRY
(data of Atwater and Benedict, 1899)

All values are average kcal/day, from 4-day experiment.

	Experiment No.					
	5	6	7	8	9	10
Heat determined	2397	3829	2434	2361	2277	2268
Protein change	−24	+40	−69	0	−21	−40
Fat change	−93	−455	−135	+266	+171	+199
Energy store change	−117	−415	−204	+266	+150	+159
Alcohol eliminated	0	0	21	0	0	8
Difference between heat estimated and observed	−4.1%	−2.7%	−1.6%	−3.2%	+1.4%	+0.7%

of the experiment proper, and then went on for his further 4 days in the calorimeter. The agreement between predicted and observed heat production becomes greater as the diet is made more uniform and easy to sample, and as the team of operators become more expert at maintaining precise temperature control. The results of Experiments 9 and 10 have not been surpassed by any investigator in this century.

At present the investigators with the greatest experience in direct calorimetry are those who deal with ruminant animals, in which loss of energy in intestinal gas invalidates measurement of metabolic rate by indirect calorimetry (Blaxter, 1971; Blaxter et al., 1972). However, modern electronic techniques have been applied to the gradient layer type of calorimeter (Benzinger et al., 1958; Spinnler et al., 1973), a water cooled garment calorimeter (Webb et al., 1972), and simple heat-sink chamber calorimeters similar to the Atwater design in which a zero heat gradient across the walls is maintained by a servo system (Garrow et al., 1977). The relative merits of different types of calorimeter are discussed in 3.2.6.

3.2.2. The respiration chamber

Atwater and Benedict (1905) described how the chamber of a direct calorimeter could be used to analyse expired air, and confirmed that heat production could be accurately predicted from measurements of oxygen consumption and carbon dioxide production. Since the heat equivalent of 1 litre of oxygen used to oxidise protein is 4.5 kcal (18.8 kJ), but to oxidise carbohydrate it yields 5.0 kcal (20.9 kJ), it is obviously necessary to correct for the nature of the substrate oxidised when converting from oxygen consumption to heat production. The ingenious formula of Weir (1949) takes advantage of the fact that the differences in energy equivalence of oxygen when burning protein, carbohydrate or fat can be offset by differences in respiratory quotient (i.e., the ratio of carbon dioxide produced to oxygen consumed) for these 3 substrates, so by his method a fairly accurate estimate of energy expenditure can be obtained by indirect calorimetry even if the catabolism of protein is not measured. Respiration chambers can provide the same amenities for long-term measurements as direct calorimeters, and they are cheaper to build. For very long-term measurements, lasting several weeks, a respiration chamber is virtually the only practicable instrument if the subject is to be provided with a reasonable amount of room and facilities for bathing. However, with large chambers there is a conflict between accuracy and the speed of response. For example the chamber being constructed in Lausanne in the department of Professor Jéquier has a volume of about 30,000 litres and is comfortably furnished. If it is ventilated at 60 l/min, it will take 500 min to change the air, so it will be some 8 h before a change in metabolism in the chamber will be detected in the outcoming air. If the oxygen consumption of the subject in the respiration chamber is 300 ml/min, the oxygen concentration in the chamber will be about 0.5% below that of the air entering the chamber. If, in order to increase the speed of response, the chamber is ventilated at 600 l/min an air change will be achieved every 50 min, but the difference in oxygen concentration between ingoing and outgoing air will be reduced to 0.05%, and will consequently be 10 times more difficult to measure accurately.

A theoretical objection to the respiration chamber is that the subject is not breathing normal air, but an atmosphere in which the oxygen concentration is already reduced and the carbon dioxide increased. In practice this does not seem to matter: Benedict and Milner showed that they obtained similar results on a subject measured on successive days with a carbon dioxide concentration of 0.03% and over 2%, although on the second day he would have probably felt breathless on exercise (Benedict, 1930).

3.2.3. Ventilated hood systems

Mouthpieces or airtight face masks can be used to collect expired air for short periods, but they are uncomfortable to use, and with untrained subjects it is difficult to avoid air leaks which would invalidate the results. Benedict (1930) described a helmet originally constructed from a galvanised iron water pail with a celluloid window, fitted over the head and sealed at the neck with a bathing cap, which proved more acceptable to patients than mouthpiece and nose clip. A more elegant version was used by Ashworth and Wolff (1969) in which the subject can rest comfortably in bed. With a paramagnetic oxygen analyser and infrared carbon dioxide analyser sampling the air sucked out of such a device it is possible to obtain both high accuracy and rapid response time in indirect calorimetry (Garrow and Hawes, 1972). Since the pressure inside the hood is always slightly below atmospheric pressure it does not matter if the neck seal leaks, provided that the leak is not so great that expired air escapes against the flow of incoming room air.

3.2.4. *The Douglas bag*

For subjects who will tolerate a mouthpiece and noseclip the Douglas bag (Douglas, 1911) provides a cheap and simple means of collecting expired air for analysis at some later time.

Courtice and Douglas (1935–6) used the method to study the effect on their metabolic rate of walking on gravel paths around the laboratory buildings. They took samples of expired air into 100-litre bags every few laps, and after ceasing exercise, and showed that the effects of a 10-mile walk persisted for several hours.

The errors in the Douglas bag technique have been critically examined by Shephard (1955). The chief sources of error are that CO_2 readily diffuses out of bags proofed with rubber, and that it is difficult to measure accurately the amount of air in a Douglas bag. Since the calculation of energy expended depends on multiplying the concentration difference between the inspired and expired air by the ventilation rate, an error of 1 litre in estimating the volume of gas in a 100-litre bag will cause an error of 1% in the answer.

3.2.5. *Portable respiration calorimeters*

The Douglas bag is clearly impractical for measuring the energy cost of certain types of work – for example that of miners at the coal face. The development of a portable respiration calorimeter by Kofranyi and Michaelis (1940) made this possible, and it is largely by the use of this "K.M." instrument that values could be assembled for the energy cost of an enormous range of human activities (Passmore and Durnin, 1955). A rather more sophisticated instrument is the integrating motor pneumotachograph, or I.M.P. (Fletcher and Wolff,

1954; Wolff, 1956). The principle in both machines is similar: the subject wears a tightly fitting mask with valves, so expired air flows to a box carried on the back. The box contains a meter which records the volume of expired air and a proportioning device so that a representative sample of this air is diverted to a small sample bag and stored for analysis at a later time. With modern plastics the problems of gas diffusion through rubber, which was a source of error with the original Douglas bags, has largely been overcome. The main difference between the K.M. and I.M.P. calorimeters is that the K.M. is a completely mechanical device, and the power to operate the proportioning pump is derived from the flow of expired air. In the I.M.P. the sampling system is self-powered, and hence it is possible to operate with a low and constant expiratory resistance, and it is also possible to adjust the sampling rate to allow longer periods of measurement. The low resistance is an important factor at high ventilation rates, since even a small increase in expiratory resistance is very noticeable to a subject at nearly maximal work rates. This may affect the energy cost of the work, which is exactly the thing which is to be measured. On the other hand, the robustness of the K.M. instrument has led to its use in many situations where high ventilation rates are not called for.

Orsini and Passmore (1951) made a comparison of the Douglas bag and K.M. methods for measuring the energy cost of carrying loads up and down stairs. They found that there was a systematic error in the meter of their K.M. instrument, which gave a value 18% too low at flow rates from 2 to 60 l/min, but since it was a constant error it could be allowed for in the calculation. Comparisons of standing and stepping exercise, measured alternately by the Douglas bag and the K.M., gave the same values within the range of physiological variation.

3.2.6. Critique of calorimetry techniques

In the previous edition of this book (Garrow, 1974b) there was a long section (pp. 64–73) about the sources of error in indirect calorimetry, and another (pp. 125–130) on the difficulties of measuring "basal" metabolism. The conclusions can be briefly summarised here, and readers wanting a fuller exposition are referred to the previous work.

Modern gas analysers are very accurate and, provided care is taken to ensure that standard gases are analysed under the same conditions of flow, temperature and humidity as the expired air, there is no reason why the actual gas analysis should be in error by more than 1%. Flow rate is more difficult to check, but in any system the accuracy can easily be checked by burning a known weight of alcohol or butane gas, to see if the result obtained by indirect calorimetry corresponds with the known thermal equivalent of the fuel. This form of calibration checks the entire system: flow rate, gas analysis and leaks. If the answer obtained agrees with the theoretical answer within 1% the system can be used with confidence, but if not, the source of error must be found.

A more important source of error, which is frequently ignored, is that measurement of resting metabolism can only be made on a patient who is at rest *and has reached a steady state*. It may be assumed that if the patient has been lying quietly for 0.5 h, and has a steady pulse rate, that this condition has been fulfilled, but this is not so, as is shown in Fig. 3.1. In a consecutive series of metabolic rate measurements made with the ventilated hood apparatus (Garrow and Hawes, 1972) on 75 patients, each measurement lasted 1 h, and the recording was started when the heart rate appeared to have become stable in the resting patient. When the record was analysed by four 15-min periods it was clear that between the first and second 0.25-h period (upper line of figure) there was a large decrease in carbon dioxide production and a smaller decrease in oxygen uptake. Between the second and third 0.25-h period the oxygen uptake had become almost stable, but carbon dioxide production was still falling, and it was only in the last two 0.25-h periods that the number of patients showing an increase or decrease in each measurement was approximately equal. This diagram illustrates that it takes about 30 min *after* the heart rate has become constant for the carbon dioxide output to become constant, so measurements of metabolic rate by indirect calorimetry, or even more so, measurements of respiratory quotient, need to be made with on-line continuous recording over a period of at least 45 min. It also shows that even when a "steady" state is achieved fluctuations of 5—10% occur from one 15-min period to the next.

36

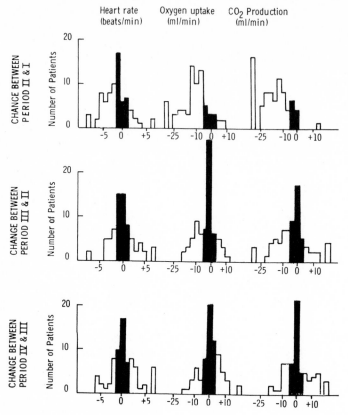

Fig. 3. 1. Changes in heart rate, oxygen uptake and carbon dioxide production in 75 patients in whom measurements were made for 4 successive periods of 15 min each.

The "resting" steady state is hard to achieve but easy to destroy. Fig. 3.2 shows part of a very long (27 h) recording of metabolic rate on a colleague during which heart rate was also being recorded. At the point indicated by the first arrow the heart recording apparatus developed a fault which might have invalidated the experiment, and it was rectified 15 min later. This transient crisis did not involve any significant physical effort on the part of the subject, but the effect of the loss of "resting" state on oxygen consumption is clear and persists for about 15 min after the fault was rectified. If continuous

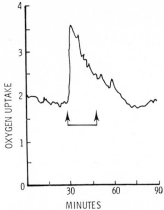

Fig. 3.2. The effect of temporary anxiety on the metabolic rate of a resting normal subject. At the point indicated by the first arrow a fault was detected in the apparatus for recording heart rate. This was rectified at the point indicated by the second arrow. Although the physical disturbance to the subject was minimal the metabolic rate was increased to nearly twice the resting value, and the resting rate was not regained for about 45 min.

recording techniques are used to monitor oxygen uptake such events are easily seen, but if the expired air is collected in a bag for later analysis an episode of this sort might well go undetected, and it would be concluded that this subject had a high resting metabolic rate.

It may be helpful to compile a rough buyers' guide to calorimeters, since there are large differences in the costs and capabilities of different types of instrument. Table 3.2 is offered to provide such a comparison, and an attempt has been made to indicate performance, based on the experience in this department where all the apparatus has been used except electromyography.

Direct calorimeters are very expensive but very accurate. The estimate of £ 5000 to £ 50,000 for cost applies to instruments which are capable of measuring heat loss to 1%, and can provide some facilities for exercise. At the lowest extreme of cost is the calorimeter described by Brown et al. (1977) which is alleged to have cost £ 100, but its performance has nothing to offer in accuracy or amenity over indirect calorimetry. At the other end of the scale is the gradient layer instru-

TABLE 3.2

RELATIVE MERITS AND LIMITATIONS OF APPARATUS DESIGNED TO MEASURE ENERGY EXPENDITURE IN MAN

Apparatus	Approx. cost (£ 1000s)	Feasible duration of measurement (h)	Range of activities measured	Detection of artefact	Approx. error in measurement (%)
Direct calorimeter	5−50	5−36	quite good	good	1
Respiration chamber	1−10	5−240	good	good	2−5
Ventilated hood	0.5−2	1−5	poor	good	2−5
Douglas bag	0.5−2	0.1−0.2	moderate	poor	2−5
Portable respirometer	0.5−2	0.2−1.0	quite good	poor	2−5
Heart rate	0.5−5	12−72	excellent	poor−good	5−10
Mechanical activity meters	0.01	infinite	good	poor	?
Electro-myography	0.5−2	?	?	poor−good	?

ment of Spinnler et al. (1973) which also has facilities for indirect calorimetry by means of a ventilated hood within the calorimeter. Without these excellent facilities it would not have been possible to do the detailed study of thermic effect and heat storage in obese and normal subjects after a glucose load (Pittet et al., 1976). The range of activities obviously depends on the size of the chamber, and the bigger the chamber the slower the response time. Our own calorimeter has a chamber similar in size to the original Atwater instrument and would cost about £ 15,000 to build now. The column in Table 3.2 "Detection of artefact" is designed to indicate how likely the operator is to be misled by false information from the instrument. With a direct calorimeter it is fairly easy to provide monitoring facilities so any dysfunction in the electronics can be easily recognised. Certainly in direct calorimetry, as in the respiration chamber, there is no doubt about what the subject is doing, or eating, or excreting, so patient artefacts are also easy to detect.

One of the advantages of the respiration chamber over the direct calorimeter is that it can be made bigger and hence acceptable for longer periods of study. The range of 5–240 h in Table 3.2 indicates that measurements less than 5 h will be inaccurate, and probably 10 days is as long as most subjects would be prepared to remain in even a luxuriously appointed cell. The accuracy of measurement for all forms of indirect calorimetry is given as 2–5%, the lower limit being set by uncertainty about the energy equivalence of oxygen (see 3.2.2). The ventilated hood, Douglas bag and portable respirometer are similar in accuracy and in price, since the cost is largely that of the gas analysis apparatus which is common to all systems in this group. The ventilated hood permits longer measurements and hence a more representative sample of expired air (see above), while the portable respirometer permits a greater range of activities. Compared with modern apparatus the Douglas bag has little to offer other than cheapness.

The remaining types of apparatus in Table 3.2 are included for comparison, but they do not provide a comparable accuracy of measurement. They are discussed further in the following sections.

To conclude this review of the techniques for indirect calorimetry, it is necessary to mention the work of Cissik et al. (1972) who suggested that an error of up to 13% might arise in indirect calorimetry in circumstances where nitrogen from a protein meal was liberated as gaseous nitrogen. However, when this work was checked by Schmid et al. (1974) and Fennessy et al. (1975) no nitrogen evolution or retention was found which might invalidate the calculations of conventional indirect calorimetry. For reasons given by Garrow (1974b) Cissik's conclusion seemed improbable, so it is a relief to have direct evidence against it.

3.2.7. Integrated electromyography

Since muscular activity is a component of energy expenditure it seems attractive to record muscle electrical activity. In the laboratory integrated electromyography is practicable (Harding and Sen, 1970), and there is a correlation between resting metabolic rate and the electromyogram (DeVries et al., 1976), suggesting that postural tone may influence the level of "resting" metabolism. However, there is so far no satisfactory method of recording muscle electrical activity to provide a convenient means of monitoring physical activity in the subject.

3.2.8. Mechanical activity monitors

Many authors have tried to record body movement as a measure of physical activity. Miller and Mumford (1967) used a pedometer, which is a weight supported on a sprung ratchet arm in such a way that a downward movement of the body (as in taking a step) imparts movement to a gear train and hence to a reading on a dial. Bloom and Eidex (1967a) mounted a timepiece on the legs of their subjects with a device which would start it when they stood up and stop it when they sat down. Greenfield and Fellner (1969) recorded the movement of lean and obese females seated in a reclining chair. All of these devices suffer from the limitation that they measure rather crudely a particular type of movement, and, particularly on fat patients, the reading of a pedometer depends as much on how it is attached to the patient as on how active the patient may be (De Looy, 1974). A much-quoted study is that of Bullen et al. (1964) who took time-lapse cine photographs of obese and non-obese girls at play in a summer camp. A total of 27,211 frames was analysed, and the level of activity of 108 obese and 52 non-obese girls was assessed. The limitation of this technique is that it can only sample a particular type of person at an organisation like a summer camp, but it is probably one of the best studies of activity.

3.2.9. Activity diaries

The most commonly used, and possibly the best available, method for measuring 24-h energy expenditure is by activity diary. The principle is simple enough: if you know the energy cost of the various activities which make up the day of the subject under study, and if you record the amount of time spent in each of these activities, then by multiplying energy cost per minute by the number of minutes spent in each activity the cost per day of that activity is known. By summing all the activities in all the minutes in the day, all the calories spent can be accounted for. The assumptions implicit in the method are:

(a) The energy cost of an activity measured (usually) by indirect calorimetry for a period of less than 15 min is representative of the cost of that activity, whatever its duration and whatever the time of day at which it occurs.

(b) The time spent in each activity during the day is not significantly altered by having to keep a record of activity.

Probably no one would claim that either assumption was entirely true; the relevant question is whether the errors involved in these assumptions are large enough to worry about. This question is best answered by making a detailed review of some of the studies which have been based on the activity diary technique.

Passmore et al. (1952) drew up a detailed energy balance sheet for 5 male students who lived in the physiology department of the University of Edinburgh for 2 weeks. During 13 consecutive days each subject recorded, from minute to minute for 16 h/day, the nature of his activity. Specially designed charts covering an 8-h period were used, with a coding system to facilitate notation, but there was provision for footnote entries for any activities not covered by the original code. For purposes of calculation, activities were grouped into 10 classes such as "light sedentary activities"; "standing at ease"; "light standing activities" and so forth. Since the experiment was designed to examine energy balance both in a relatively sedentary and in a strenuous way of life, the first 3 days were spent indoors and fairly inactive, during the next 5 days track walking (or when it was too wet, stair climbing) was included in the routine, and for the last 5 days the subjects reverted to their former sedentary pursuits. The subjects walked 10–15 miles/day at a speed of 4.2–4.8 miles/h. All food eaten during the experiment was recorded, and the energy content of the food was measured by analysis of duplicate samples. The energy cost of each activity was determined by indirect calorimetry with a K.M. machine for a period of 6–15 min. The final calculation of energy balance for the 13-day period is shown in Table 3.3.

TABLE 3.3

TOTAL ESTIMATED ENERGY EXPENDITURE (by intermittent indirect calorimetry) AND INTAKE OF 5 SUBJECTS STUDIED FOR 13 DAYS BY PASSMORE ET AL. (1952)

	John	George	Alistair	Evan	Ian
Weight (kg)	59.4	69.1	75.5	79.6	83.1
Estimated expenditure (kcal)	34,310	51,510	45,980	46,000	49,580
Estimated intake (kcal)	36,280	53,090	51,020	48,130	46,300
Estimated imbalance	+1970	+1580	+5040	+2130	−3280
Weight change (kg)	+0.34	+0.31	+2.66	+0.14	−2.49
kcal/kg weight change	5800	5100	1900	15,300	1300
Imbalance as % intake	+5.4	+2.8	+10.0	+4.4	−7.1
Average intake per day (kcal)	2800	4080	3930	3700	3480

The authors conclude that the agreement between the estimates of intake and expenditure was "satisfactory" and suggest that the technique might be used to estimate the energy expenditure of operatives, especially those engaged in heavy industry.

This is an important publication from a laboratory renowned for its contributions in the field of human energy measurements, so it is necessary to examine closely the basis for their conclusions. Certainly estimates of input and output agree within a few percent, and the imbalance is in the direction which would be suggested by the weight change of the subject. However, when the weight change is related to the magnitude of the energy imbalance the result, in kcal/kg, shows very large variations. As the authors themselves state "it is impossible to estimate how far these differences (in weight) represent changes in body tissue". Dole et al. (1955) showed that, in obese subjects, alternating cycles of over- and underfeeding produced changes in labile tissue which apparently had an energy value of about 2500 kcal (10.7 MJ) per kg, so one might have expected a value of about this magnitude for the weight changes in Passmore's subjects. Another criticism is that the strenuous exercise which was chosen for these subjects was track walking, because it was "hardwork, a steady and continuous exercise, whose metabolic cost can easily be determined". Indeed the 3 activities of track walking (or stair climbing if it was too wet), lying in bed, and "light sedentary activities" between them account for 63–74% of the total energy expenditure of these subjects, and of these three the "light sedentary activities" was the greatest energy user in all but one subject, who was ill and spent several days in bed. Thus the general agreement between estimated input and output does not necessarily show that a similar study on operatives in heavy industry would be reliable.

Another classical study using the activity diary technique is that of Edholm et al. (1955) who measured the energy intake and output of 12 military cadets for a period of 2 weeks. In this publication the values for individual subjects performing the same task show a wide variation: for example the energy cost of lying was 1.86 kcal/min for one subject (mean of 3 measurements), while for another it was 1.18 kcal/min (mean of 7 measurements). Similarly the range for sitting was 1.34–2.06 kcal/min in different individuals, for standing 1.43–2.20, and for marching at the regulation pace of 3.4 miles/h the range was 4.53–7.34 kcal/min. On average the cadets spent 17 h 41 min/day either lying, sitting or standing. Thus the measurement of these low levels of activity is the chief factor which determines the accuracy of the whole estimate of energy expenditure. In 3.2.5 we have already discussed the errors inherent in estimating the energy cost of lying from a short period of indirect calorimetry: these errors are relevant to activity diary techniques, since if the estimated cost per minute is wrong the integrated cost over a longer period will be correspondingly wrong, even if the duration of the activity is correctly recorded.

The second assumption underlying the activity diary technique is that the time spent in each activity is not significantly affected by having to keep an activity record. This is another untestable assumption: probably for the military cadets, whose activity was in any case fairly closely regimented, the assumption would be valid. However, for less disciplined subjects the keeping of an accurate activity diary is a major undertaking. Anyone who doubts this should try the experiment himself: the recording of activity does not become automatic, but requires constant vigilance. In practice either the subject tends to adopt a pattern of activity which is easy to record, or else he forgets for longer or shorter periods and makes his entries as a series of recalls. Personally I find that keeping an activity diary with reasonable accuracy for 2 or 3 days is sufficient to reduce me to a state of exasperation.

It may be argued that if the activity diary is an accurate record for the duration of the experiment it does not matter that there may be differences between the activity recorded and habitual activity. Unfortunately it does matter, since the period of observation is necessarily short. If, therefore, during the period of observation the level of activity (or of food intake for that matter) is significantly changed, the observations are being made in an unsteady state and changes in body composition are likely to occur and invalidate any estimate of energy balance.

The activity diary technique is capable of endless modification by which social acceptability is gained at the expense of accuracy. The most tedious part of the method used by Passmore et al. (1952) and Edholm et al. (1955) in the studies quoted above is the calibration of each subject for oxygen consumed at each task. It is much easier to consult the comprehensive tables of Passmore and Durnin (1955) and to assume that each subject has the energy requirements which the tables say he should have for each task. Since the variation between individuals covers roughly a 2-fold range this assumption will often be wrong by 20% or more. For some purposes this level of inaccuracy is quite acceptable: a supplies officer victualling an expedition of, say, 20 men would do very well if he estimated their requirements within 20%, and since some of the errors for some individuals will be on the high side, and some will be too low, the party as a whole should be adequately catered for by reference to group averages such as those in Passmore and Durnin's excellent review. However, when it comes to trying to track down the small cumulative error which leads to obesity such errors are totally unacceptable and make nonsense of the whole investigation. For example Stefanik et al. (1959) classified the activities of 14 obese and 14 non-obese boys into "light", "moderate" or "very active" according to whether the particular occupation came below, between or above two arbitrary thresholds of 150 kcal (0.63 MJ) per h and 250 kcal (1.05 MJ) per h in the energy expenditure tables. Using this blunt instrument they were unable to detect a significant difference between obese and non-obese, and it would have been amazing had they done so. McCarthy (1966) used a still more approximate approach: she asked the Trinidadian women to recall how much of the previous 24 h had been spent lying, sitting, in light exercise or in moderate-to-heavy work. She concluded that "Based solely on time spent at activities (probably an inadequate index), the obese group was as active as the control group."

It is interesting that the investigator with the least accurate data is somewhat firmer in his conclusions. "In this study, physical activity levels of the more obese groups were not lower than those of the less obese groups." Thus concluded Lincoln (1972) who asked his subjects, by mail, if their physical activity on the job was a great deal, quite a bit, a little, or hardly any, and if their hours per week in exercise were none, 2–5, or 6 or over. There is something rather charming about so innocent an approach.

3.2.10. Methods based on heart rate recording

In the previous edition of this book (Garrow, 1974b) pp. 79–84 were concerned with a review of the technique and limitations of heart rate recording as a means of monitoring energy expenditure. A recent and comprehensive review of this topic has been made by Warnold and Lenner (1977), so only the main points will be summarised here.

The advantage of this technique to measure energy expenditure is that it can be applied to a very large range of activities (in fact almost anything that does not involve immersion in water), measurements can be made over long periods, and the process of measurement has little effect on the pattern of activity of the subject. If you are wearing a well designed heart rate monitor it is easy to forget its presence completely, which is more than can be said for any of the other devices listed in Table 3.2 except, perhaps, for the pedometer. The duration of measurement is given as 12–72 h, since unfamiliarity with the apparatus will probably invalidate measurements in the first few hours, and 72 h is about the maximum time for which electrodes will function satisfactorily, and it is important to use an electrode jelly which preserves good electrical contact without ulcerating the skin (De Looy and James, 1972). Detection of artefact may be poor or good, depending on the associated electronics, which also explains the large price range shown in Table 3.2. The simplest apparatus is a SAMI (Baker et al., 1967) which detects the R wave in the electro-cardiogram and uses this to trigger the release of a minute charge into an electrochemical cell: this has the effect of driving silver from one electrode to the other. To play back the information a current is passed in the reverse direction through the cell until all the silver is back where it started. This simple device is very prone to artefact, so more sophisticated apparatus can be used to detect the R wave and record the heart rate. Warnold and Lenner used apparatus which recognised the slope, amplitude and width of the R wave, and had automatic gain control, so the signal was maintained at adequate size. The output was either telemetered or fed directly to a small portable tape recorder.

However elaborate the electronics may be, it is necessary for the user to be aware of the limitations of this technique. It is essential that good electrode contact should be maintained, and it is wise to inspect the ECG signal at least daily to ensure that it is of good quality and not obscured by noise. Having obtained a reliable record of heart rate the problem remains of converting this to energy expenditure. In general there is a good relationship between heart rate and metabolic rate, but the regression of one on the other differs in different individuals, and in the same individual in different postures (Booyens and Hervey, 1960). Also the relationship can be upset by severe psychological stress: Moss and Wynar (1970) report an increase in heart rate from 73 to 154 beats/min in junior doctors presenting cases for criticism. Despite these limitations heart rate remains a good indicator of oxygen consumption, as is illustrated in Fig. 3.3. This shows a part of a continuous recording of both heart rate and oxygen consumption in a subject at rest in a ventilated hood (Garrow and Hawes, 1972). Between 2 a.m. and 4 a.m. she was asleep, and the minor changes in oxygen uptake with changing levels of sleep are well reflected in the heart rate recording. Later on the same day she was propped up in bed watching the Apollo 14 moon landing on a television set. The generally higher heart rate is partly due to the change in posture, and the minor physical disturbance of blood and urine sampling, and the excitement of the moon landing, are both shown on the oxygen and heart rate traces.

The problem of relating heart rate to metabolic rate has been reviewed by Goldsmith et al. (1966), Bradfield (1971) and Warnold and Lenner (1977). During fairly vigorous exercise, when the heart rate is over 90 beats/min, the correlation between the two variables is high, but in resting subjects the heart rate may vary between 60 and 80 beats/min with little change in metabolic rate. Thus it is necessary to make two calibration lines for each subject (Warnold and Lenner, 1977), one for active, and another for sedentary periods, and these have different slopes, so at about 80 beats/min it is not certain if the upper end of the "sedentary" line, or the lower end of the "active" line, should be used.

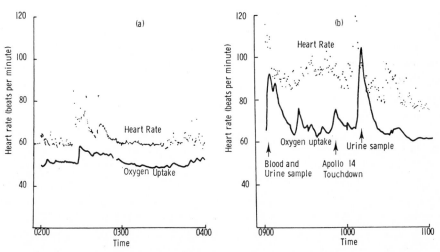

Fig. 3.3. The relationship of heart rate to oxygen consumption in one subject (a) between the hours of 02.00 and 04.00 while asleep and fasting, (b) between the hours of 09.00 and 11.00, sitting, watching television.

3.3. The relationship of energy intake, and of physical activity, to obesity

Garrow (1974b) reviewed 13 publications, covering a total of 1481 subjects, in which weight, intake and/or physical activity were measured, and failed to find any convincing evidence that in general obese people ate more, or exercised less, than thin people. It was concluded that the errors in the methods used to measure energy intake, energy expenditure, and physical activity were so large that they were incapable of detecting the small imbalance between intake and output which is necessary to cause obesity. An excellent review of studies on energy balance in man over the past 25 years has recently been published by Edholm (1977).

One investigation which was not covered by the previous review was that of Mayer et al. (1956), in which they studied workers in a jute mill in West Bengal. They concluded that "caloric intake increases with activity only within a certain zone ("normal activity"). Below that range ("sedentary activity") a decrease in activity is not followed by a decrease in food intake but, on the contrary, by an increase. Body weight is also increased in that zone. The picture is similar to that found in experimental animals." This conclusion is often quoted in support of the idea that below a certain critical level of physical activity the system for controlling energy balance breaks down, and certainly the theory is an attractive one. The publication is important because it seems to show a definite cause for obesity, which is refreshing after so many inconclusive papers. It is therefore important to make a critical examination of the original data, especially as they bear on the range of sedentary activity. Body weight and energy intake are only given as averages in graphical form, so the data in Table 3.4 have been obtained by measurement from the published figure.

The first 3 occupation groups are classified as "sedentary", and the next 4 as "light work". It is then observed that the sedentary group is heavier, and eats more, than the light work group, hence the conclusion quoted above. However, this conclusion depends entirely on the arbitrary occupation groups, and it appears that there is an arithmetical error in the calculation of the average weight for the

TABLE 3.4

BODY WEIGHT, ENERGY INTAKE AND PHYSICAL ACTIVITY AMONG
JUTE WORKERS IN WEST BENGAL (data of Mayer et al., 1956)

Occupation	n	Average weight (lb)	Energy intake (kcal/day)
Stallholders	13	168	3300
Supervisors	8	142	3400
Clerks (on premises, no sport)	22	109	3200
Clerks (commute over 3 miles)	13	124	2700
Clerks (commute over 6 miles)	10	120	2700
Clerks (commute and soccer)	5	110	2800
Mechanics (few power aids)	22	112	2600

sedentary group. It can easily be verified from Table 3.4 that the average weight of the individuals in the sedentary group is about 133 lb, and the value of 139 lb which is shown in the original paper is incorrect. If it were not for the 13 stallholders and 8 supervisors (for whom no direct evidence of physical activity is given) the data seem to show an even stranger phenomenon: clerks who live on the company premises and do not partake in sport eat about 400 kcal/day more, and weigh about 12 lb less, than clerks who commute daily to work over many miles, or play soccer. It is the stallholders and supervisors who are responsible for the alleged association of obesity and inactivity, and it seems at least as reasonable to ascribe their weight to the fact that they had access to a better diet as to their inactivity, especially as inactivity does not seem to have prevented the sedentary clerks from maintaining a low body weight on a high energy intake.

So far as I know the observations of Mayer et al. (1956) have not been confirmed by any other investigation in man, but an interesting test of the theory that very low levels of physical activity are associated with increased food intake can be made by examining the results of Warnold and Lenner (1977). They studied young diabetic men and women for periods of 7 days during which they were "extremely inactive", and then for 7—11 days in "normal light activity", so it might be expected from the conclusion of Mayer et al.

(1956) that they would overeat in the "extremely inactive" phase. In fact this was not found: the ratio of intake to expenditure was not significantly different in the two phases.

We can therefore summarise the present situation by saying that although many workers have measured energy intake and output on many groups of subjects, the nature of the energy imbalance in obesity is still unknown. This situation is not too surprising if we consider the nature of the problem in quantitative terms. From the data discussed above it is clear that within groups of individuals the coefficient of variation of energy intake or expenditure is about 15%. Thus a range of ±30% from the mean will cover about 95% of the group, and if there are more than 40 individuals in the group there will be about a 2-fold difference between the requirements of the lowest and the highest member.

Let us, for simplicity of calculation, postulate 3 separate communities, each with a similar and homogeneous population, and with a mean energy requirement of 3000 kcal/day. In village A all the inhabitants maintain constant weight throughout the year, but in villages B and C all the inhabitants become steadily more obese, and each one increases in weight by 5 kg/year by laying down adipose tissue which contains 3.3 kg fat and 1.7 kg water. In all other respects the body composition of the inhabitants of villages B and C remain constant. However in village B they all eat exactly the same amount as in A, but expend less energy, whereas in village C they expend exactly the same amount of energy as in village A but they eat more. Consider now the task of a nutritionist who was called upon to explain the cause of obesity in villages B and C.

If dietary surveys of great accuracy were done in all 3 villages the distribution of intakes would be as indicated by the continuous line in Fig. 3.4A, B and C, for the 3 villages. Equally accurate estimates of energy expenditure would yield the distribution indicated by the dotted curves. In village A the curves for intake and expenditure coincide, but in B and C they are displaced by 84 kcal/day, since a cumulative error of 84 kcal/day will amount to 30,000 kcal in a year, which is equivalent to 5 kg of extra adipose tissue.

The hypothetical problem set out above is far easier to solve than that which nutritionists encounter in real life. Obese people do not

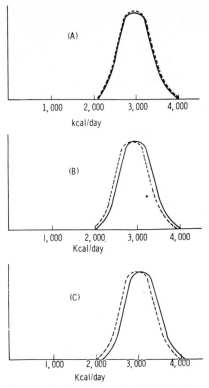

Fig. 3.4. Comparison of intake (———) and expenditure (————) in the inhabitants of 3 hypothetical villages. The inhabitants of village A maintain constant weight, but those of B and C gain 5 kg/year.

live in separate communities and behave in a uniform and predictable way. They do not all gain weight at a constant rate: some may be obese and currently losing weight, while other people who are currently lean may be gaining. Even if obese people are, over a year, gaining 5 kg there is no reason to suppose that they will gain *pro rata* for a short period of investigation; indeed there is every reason to believe that a period of intensive dietary investigation would be atypical rather than typical of the year as a whole.

3.4. Summary: the gap between what is required in the measurement of energy intake and expenditure and what is possible by available techniques

Within homogeneous groups of normal people there is about a 2-fold difference between the requirements at the lowest and the highest end of the range. The reason for this large variation between individuals is not understood, but it is established beyond all reasonable doubt that a range of this magnitude exists.

Energy intake and expenditure can be measured by various techniques which have been reviewed in this chapter. Each method has its advantages and disadvantages, but in general the more accurate the technique the more trouble it involves for both investigator and subject. Thus the universal uncertainty principle applies: the more confident you may be in the precision of the result the less sure you can be that the measured value for energy intake or expenditure is a true reflection of the habitual intake or expenditure of the subject. It is necessary that the normal energy equilibrium of the subject should be upset as little as possible by the investigation, since changes in body composition can otherwise invalidate energy balance studies.

The magnitude of the error in energy balance which will lead to severe and rapidly developing obesity is small compared to the range of variation of energy intake and expenditure within a group of individuals. To take a very favourable example: if the coefficient of variation of requirements within a group is 15%, and the balance error leading to obesity is 3%, it can be shown that on statistical grounds alone it would be necessary to do accurate energy balance studies on at least 200 subjects to detect this magnitude of error.

Obese people become obese because their energy intake is too high, or their output is too low, but present techniques are inadequate to enable us to say which explanation, or what combination of the two, is the most correct in any given obese individual.

CHAPTER 4

Factors affecting energy intake

Four years ago the "dual centre" concept dominated research on the regulation of food and water intake, and there was an impressive body of experimental work to support it. In the hypothalamus there were two regions which had powerful effects on feeding behaviour: the lateral and the ventromedial nuclei were labelled in undergraduate textbooks the "hunger centre" and the "satiety centre" respectively. Bilateral lesions of the ventromedial nucleus in rats caused the animals to eat voraciously and become obese (Kennedy, 1950). However, rats with a lesion in the lateral hypothalamus were indifferent to food and, unless fed, might die of starvation.

All this is still true, but the dual centre theory has had its anatomical foundations undermined by recent research, and some of the superstructure has collapsed under critical attack. In revising this chapter it is easy to catalogue new doubts about the control mechanism for food intake, but difficult to offer alternative theories which will fit the new observations. The reader who wants an expert assessment of the current state of knowledge would do well to consult two recent conference reports: "Appetite and food intake", edited by T. Silverstone, a conference held in Berlin in December 1975, and published by Dahlem Konferenzen; and "Hunger, basic mechanisms and clinical implications" edited by D. Novin, W. Wyrwicka and G. Bray, a conference held in Los Angeles in January 1975, and published by Raven Press.

4.1. The role of the hypothalamus in controlling food intake

The rise and fall of the dual centre theory of appetite control have been well described by Grossman (1976). The classical observations of the early neuroanatomists are still true and reproducible: this is no case of scientific fraud or incompetence, but these theories have had to be extended in the light of new knowledge, just as Einstein's work revised and extended Newton's cosmology which had until then served very well. The dual centre theory became unusable when Gold (1973) showed that the ventromedial nucleus was irrelevant to satiety: precise knifecut lesions showed that the ventromedial hyperphagic syndrome depended on damage to nearby ventral noradrenergic tracts. The lateral hypothalamic nucleus cannot be regarded as the seat of the hunger sensation, since destruction of the nucleus produces a profound decrease in general activation which includes total lack of interest in food. However, "recovered lateral" rats (who have been nursed through this period of apathy) regain the ability to maintain body weight, although their responses to feeding stimuli are still somewhat abnormal (Wolgin et al., 1976). More remarkable still, cats with a lateral hypothalamic lesion are actually *stimulated* to eat by a dose of amphetamine which would normally *stop* a cat eating (Wolgin et al., 1976). Other non-specific methods of arousing the animal, such as pinching its tail, will make the lesioned animal eat.

The shift, therefore, has been away from viewing the hypothalamus as generator of signals to start and stop eating, and towards a view of it as a place where nerve fibres bring together many interacting signals. The problem now is to understand how the circuits are laid, and whence and whither the signals travel. Russek (1976) has proposed a mathematical model by which if the concentration of glucagon, insulin, adrenalin and glucose in the blood, the liver glycogen, the rate of utilization of glucose by the lateral hypothalamus, body weight and osmolarity, and air temperature are known, and if all these are entered into the equation, food intake can be predicted. The constants in the formula need not concern us now: the point is that these are the main factors to which the hypothalamic control system is known to respond. There is still room for a modified version of control systems based on temperature (Brobeck, 1948), or blood glucose (Mayer, 1953; Mayer and Arees, 1968), or something which senses the total fat content of the animal (Kennedy, 1953, 1966).

The hypothalamus certainly has relevance to food intake in man. Obesity due to hypothalamic damage is rare but well documented:

Bray and Gallagher (1975) give an extensive review and report 8 cases. The daring stereotactic exploits of Quaade (1974) have shown that direct stimulation of the lateral hypothalamus in man can cause powerful sensations of hunger. However, hypothalamic damage is one of the very rare causes of obesity, and to understand even that we need to know more about the source of the signals which the hypothalamus receives.

4.2. Intestinal factors affecting food intake

The fashion for equating hunger with gastric motility waned when Bloom et al. (1970) and Stunkard and Fox (1971) were unable to show any strong association between the two. However, the interest in the gut as a source of satiety signals revived when Leibling et al. (1975) showed that the presence of food in the duodenum of a rat with a gastric fistula stopped the rat from feeding. They further linked the satiety response to the release of the gut hormone cholecystokinin and have now shown that when this hormone is infused into rhesus monkeys the meal size is reduced in proportion to the amount of hormone given. Certain amino acids, notably L-phenylalanine (but not D-phenylalanine) are potent releasers of the hormone, and have corresponding satiating effects in these monkeys (Gibbs and Smith, 1977).

Evidently gut hormones are not the only messengers coming from the intestine and reducing food intake after a meal. Feeding in the rat is inhibited by infusion of glucose into the stomach or duodenum or hepatic portal vein (Booth and Jarman, 1976). The nature of the diet may also affect the concentration of neurotransmitters in the brain: specifically it has been shown that there is a relationship between tryptophan in the diet and serotonin synthesis in the rat brain (Wurtman and Fernstrom, 1975). However, the relevance of all these possible ways in which the brain might receive satiety signals from the gut is still not established in man.

It has been suggested by human physiologists that the energy density of food might affect intake of total energy. Heaton (1973) postulates that food fibre may limit intake, and Hunt et al. (1975) that dilution of food with water would delay gastric emptying and hence increase satiety, but one test of this theory has failed to support it (Durrant et al., 1977).

4.3. Endocrine factors affecting food intake

This topic has been well reviewed by Bray (1974). Insulin increases food intake, either when given acutely or over a long time, but not in rats with a lesion in their lateral hypothalamus. Hypophysectomy decreases food intake, but hypophysectomised rats will still overeat and become obese if they have lesions in their ventromedial hypothalamus. In hypophysectomised rats growth hormone will increase food intake. Glucagon and estrogens both decrease food intake, and castration in female rats promotes weight gain.

4.4. Integration of the factors controlling food intake in man

There is no shortage of factors which can be shown to influence food intake in one model system or another. To understand energy balance in man we need to know how the control system is integrated, and why the human race tends more often than most species to err in the direction of a positive balance with consequent obesity.

4.4.1. The big head problem

At 8.30 a.m. on Tuesday 25th October 1977 Dr. George Cahill started to give one of the best review lectures I have heard in my life. It will appear in the proceedings of the Second International Congress of Obesity, edited by G. Bray, but is unpublished as this is written. The topic was obesity and diabetes, and the final passage was one of these brilliant syntheses of which few speakers are capable: Dr. Cahill identified a major metabolic dilemma with which man is confronted, which he called the "big head problem". Cahill expressed it better, but basically it is this. Man has a big brain with a power consumption of about 20 W, and it cannot use fatty acids as fuel, but only glucose, glycerol or ketone bodies. This is a severe disadvantage in time of famine, when fuel from the body fat is mostly in the form of fatty acid, and it can be argued that in this situation the maturity onset diabetic has an advantage. However, the point which is relevant to the control of energy balance in non-diabetic man is that the intellectual advantage which the big brain gives to man is that he is not at the mercy of the factors reviewed in previous sections to determine food intake. The equation of Russek (1976) is complex, but takes no account of intelligence, and therefore does not describe the mechanism controlling food intake in man. Primitive man, about to set out on a long sea voyage, or knowing that the harvest season was nearly over, would have the wit to eat while there was food available in anticipation of future hunger. It is characteristic of the higher animals, such as primates, that their intake of food is less predictable, since higher cortical activity often overrides hypothalamic signals (Anand, 1974). It is only in the higher Douc monkeys, gibbons and chimpanzees that food sharing has been observed (Kavanagh, 1972), which is another possibility not catered for in Russek's equation.

Booth et al. (1976) have demonstrated that in man satiety is a learned response. Volunteers were given a disguised preload of starch immediately before a sandwich lunch, with a high or low preload (65 or 5 g) associated with distinctive flavours, and after a few days they learned to eat less after the larger preload. When this response was established the flavour associated with high and low energy preloads were reversed, and on the first test day the meal was appropriate in size to the *flavour* of the preload on which the subjects had been trained, but wrong for the *energy* content of the preload actually taken. After a few days the (now wrong) learned response was extinguished. It is hard to explain these results on any basis other than that advanced by the authors, namely that satiety is a learned response, and in this case associated with a particular flavour. This response has been confirmed and can be demonstrated also in rats (Booth, 1977). It should not be thought that man alone eats more than is good for him: by any reasonable standards the rat will shorten his life by overeating if he gets a chance (Ross and Bras, 1975), and "the longevity of rats permitted freedom of dietary choice can be predicted accurately solely on the basis of their dietary behaviour and growth responses early in life" (Ross et al., 1976).

The complexity of human eating behaviour is matched by the deviousness of investigators in this field. Nisbett (1968) and Schachter (1968) went to great lengths to mislead their subjects concerning the nature of the experiment in which they were participating, and were able to show that many nutritionally irrelevant factors, like the supposed time of day or anxiety about receiving an electric shock, affected food intake. It was at first suggested that this sensitivity to "external" influences was a characteristic of obese people, and lean people paid more attention to true physiological signals of hunger, or "internal" stimuli. This has not been confirmed, and on average the moderately obese seem to be more "external" than either lean or very obese people (Rodin et al., 1977b) but there is great variation within each weight group.

Perhaps the ultimate in deviousness is the report by Pudel and Oetting (1977) which is dedicated to Dr. J.-E. Meyer. The workers in Goettingen study the amount of a liquid food which their subjects suck from a cylinder at a meal, but of course the apparatus is so designed that the food which the subject is actually taking is coming from a hidden reservoir, while the liquid which he sees disappearing from the cylinder in front of him as he sucks is in fact being pumped away to waste. The investigators can thus alter the ratio of the amount of food which the subject thinks he is taking to the amount he actually takes. So far this is routine psychiatric trickery, but the new twist comes when the investigators now explain the trick of the "refilling bowl" to the subject. Pudel and Oetting (1977) report the fascinating result: normal subjects who had been fooled into eating more by the refilling bowl no longer do so when the trick is explained, obese subjects who formerly ate much more from the refilling bowl still overeat when the trick is explained, but to a lesser extent, while a group called "latent obese" actually eat less than in the control period when the trick is explained, although previously they ate about the same amount as the non-obese controls.

The situation is indeed complex if we must distinguish at least 3 groups: the lean who are naturally lean, the obese who are naturally obese, and the lean who are naturally obese, but manage to remain of normal weight by restrained eating. This concept of restrained eaters has been developed by Herman and Polivy (1975), Herman and Mack (1975) and Hibscher and Herman (1977). This is the size of Cahill's "big head problem" in human obesity. Even before we come to consider the effects of society, gastronomy, illness or upbringing it is very difficult to interpret the results of laboratory feeding experiments in man. Even if we knew exactly the neurophysiology of the hypothalamus, and the neural and endocrine signals which it receives, there is little reason to suppose that the effect of these signals would be seen in eating behaviour in man after the monstrous bureaucracy of his intellect has scrambled the message.

4.4.2. The social problem and gastronomy

It can be argued that the previous section exaggerated the role of the brain in overriding the natural physiological signals which might otherwise regulate energy balance. After all, man can override his temperature control system also: he may take sauna baths, or wear clothes which are fashionable rather than appropriate to the ambient temperature, but he still maintains a body temperature close to 37°C. However, food intake is a different case from thermoregulation, since food has an important social function as well as a nutritive one. What, when and how much we eat is largely conditioned by the society in which we live. This is easily shown if the food habits of different ethnic groups are compared (De Garine, 1972). In different places food has every kind of significance: to establish social status, to placate enemies, as religious symbols or to bind together communities. Nor does this apply only to distant countries and backward tribes. In every community the national cuisine is an important feature, hence the restaurants advertising characteristic national dishes in every capital city in the world.

The importance of flavour goes far beyond providing variety for the sophisticated palate. Rozin (1976) points out that many of the most sought foods are "unpalatable" in that children or people unaccustomed to them find them unpleasant: chili pepper, which is a mainstay of adult Mexican cuisine, is used in some Mexican villages applied to the mother's breast to promote weaning. It is important that some foods should be recognised as wholesome and distinguished from those which are poisonous. It is well documented that rats who have been poisoned will starve rather than eat food with a similar flavour even if it is not poisoned, and this characteristic of bait-shyness must be important to the survival of communities.

Within communities obesity is related to social class. In New York and London obesity is commoner in the lower social classes (Gold-blatt et al., 1965; Silverstone et al., 1969; Ashwell and Etchell, 1974; Baird et al., 1974b). In Germany Pflanz (1962) reported that obesity was commoner in lower social class women (as in other affluent societies) but that in German men the rule was reversed: this must mean that it is socially more acceptable for men to be overweight in Germany. In less affluent countries like India obesity is generally commoner in the upper social classes (Gour and Gupta, 1968), presumably since the poor have limited access to food, and stoutness implies success.

The relationship between obesity and taste responsiveness has been widely researched. Cabanac et al. (1971) found that normal people develop an aversion to sweet drinks after a glucose load, while obese people do not. Rodin (1975) tested Yale University undergraduates with 5 milkshakes of varying sweetness and found no difference in preference between the normal weight and overweight subjects, but the overweight students were prepared to work harder at a puzzle to obtain the flavour of milkshake they preferred. An interesting aspect of this study was that the weight of the students was known over the previous two years, and if it had been stable without conscious effort on the part of the student this weight was assumed to be the "set point" for that student. It was part of the hypothesis of Cabanac et al. (1971) that people below their set point were relatively insensitive to physiological cues, but this view is not supported by the results of Rodin (1975). Other investigators (Underwood et al., 1973; Thompson et al., 1976) have obtained much less clearcut differences in taste response than those reported by Cabanac and Duclaux (1970) but in general confirm that obese subjects find sweet taste pleasanter than do lean subjects. If the only food available is monotonous but available in unlimited quantity subjects will become bored and take less of it whether they are obese (Hashim and Van Itallie, 1965; Campbell et al., 1971) or not (Cabanac and Rabe, 1976).

Wooley et al. (1976) report differences between lean and obese people in salivation (and by implication appetite) when presented with pizza. Lean subjects salivated more at the sight of the pizza if they had not recently eaten than if they had recently eaten, but in the obese subjects this was not so. When the obese subjects were food deprived but did not expect to eat the pizza they salivated less, while in these conditions the lean subjects salivated more. It is not clear how these results should be interpreted, but at least it is clear that previous diet, expectation and palatability all interact in the control of food intake in man. This will become increasingly important as the human race becomes more urbanised. It is now quite rare in affluent countries for men to subsist on food they have produced: for various technical and economic reasons most food is now commercially processed before it is eaten, and there is every reason to believe that this trend will increase. Food technology is now so advanced that the taste, appearance and texture of processed food may resemble that of a natural food, but the nutritive content of the processed food may bear no resemblance to its natural analogue (Yudkin, 1963).

4.4.3. The effects of drugs and illness

Another important respect in which man differs from laboratory animals is that he takes drugs, either as a treatment for illness, or for specific pharmacological effects. Of course laboratory animals, which are used as models for studying the control of food intake, may also become ill, but in this event reputable workers would discard them as inappropriate. This is understandable but not very logical, since man, the species being modelled, is not "discarded" when ill, but treated with drugs or surgery which may have profound effects on food intake. It is noticeable that when workers allow laboratory rats a choice of foods and wait until they die from natural causes (Ross et al., 1976), their control of food intake is as fallible as that in man.

In man, physical or mental illness is a common cause of anorexia (Hawkins, 1976). Bypass surgery (Bray et al., 1976a) and cancer (DeWys, 1977) decrease food intake and alter taste sensitivity, and chemotherapy for cancer is very often associated with loss of appetite. In addition to the anorexia which is an unwanted side effect of drug therapy for disease, there is the extensive use of drugs specifically to induce anorexia: in Britain the cost to the National Health Service of drugs to treat obesity by reducing food intake was £ 2.5m in 1973 and had increased to £ 3.5m by 1975, which is the latest year for which figures are available.

Cigarette smoking is associated with weight change (Khosla and Lowe, 1971, 1972; Comstock and Stone, 1972; Garvey et al., 1974), but Ashwell and North (1978) have shown that there is an interesting interaction between smoking and social class in the effect on obesity. Higher social class smoking men were more obese than non-smokers of similar social class, while among lower social class men the smokers were leaner than the non-smokers. Among upper social class women there was no significant difference in obesity between smokers and non-smokers, but in lower social class women non-smokers were more obese than smokers.

Weight gain is a side effect of several drugs. The effects of the contraceptive pill on weight are variable, and it is not clear if it has a specific effect on food intake, but significant weight gain is associated with taking alcohol (Pequignot et al., 1973), antidepressants (Paykel et al., 1973) and marihuana (Greenberg et al., 1976).

4.4.4. Childhood influences

The question of early onset obesity is discussed in Chapter 7, but we may note here that apart from any question of fat cell size and number there is impressive evidence that control of food intake is a skill taught in childhood (Garrow, 1976). Bruch (1940) noted that obese children are overfed and overprotected, and could not be expected to recognise the signs of genuine hunger because they were never allowed to experience it. On the contrary, they were taught to associate food with consolation for every kind of misfortune except the need for food, so it was understandable that their control of food intake was erratic. This fact is rediscovered from time to time by succeeding generations of child psychologists.

It is impressive that the influence of the mother on teaching the young what kind and quantity of food to eat is seen in many species: this subject is excellently reviewed by Wyrwicka (1976). The potency of maternal example is illustrated in an experiment in which a normal cat was separated from her kittens and persuaded (by stimulation of brain electrodes) to prefer eating banana rather than meat, which is the natural preference of cats. When a kitten, who had expressed the normal preference for meat elsewhere, was put in the cage with the mother cat the kitten did not eat meat, but the banana which the mother cat ate. This remarkable study shows how difficult it is to distinguish between genetic and environmental influences in the feeding behaviour of young animals. Ounstead and Sleigh (1975) conclude that there are "powerful self-regulatory controls within the infant" which determine how much milk it will take from a bottle, and during recovery from malnutrition children switch off their burst of catch-up growth when they reach the appropriate weight for their height (Ashworth, 1974).

An interesting speculation, which does not seem to have been pursued, is that of Hall (1975). The composition of human breast milk (and that of other mammals) changes during the feed, and it is quite likely that this is an important factor in teaching the child to recognise where it is in the course of a feed at the breast. If this is so the bottle-fed baby is at a disadvantage, since it has a milk of constant composition and flavour, and is thus deprived of any landmarks to help him navigate in this difficult area.

4.4.5. Where are the set points?

At the meeting on "Energy balance in man" in Paris in 1971 it was implicit in every presentation concerning the mechanism controlling food intake that somewhere there was a reference value, or "set point", on which the control system tended to converge. There were differences in concept about the nature of this value, and the terminology varied (La Magnen used "set point", Cabanac "consign value of body weight", Shapiro "an ideal mass of adipose tissue", Quaade "preferred weight", Miller "predetermined weight") but all agreed that there was a fixed reference value of something, without which the system would lose all stability. When, following the paper by

Shapiro (1973), I challenged this shibboleth the assembled experts rebuked me. Indeed it was probably that experience which stimulated me to write the first edition of this book.

Today the set point lobby is still strong: for example the predictive equation of Russek (1976) invokes hepatic glucoreceptors to modulate the rate of food intake, but still relies on a weight set point for long-term stability in his model, otherwise it would drift as energy output changed. Faust et al. (1977) postulate a fat cell size as a set point with reference to which food intake is regulated. However, some heavy artillery is now shooting in the other direction: thus Booth (1976) says "Not one set point comparator system has to my knowledge been unambiguously identified anywhere in physiology or human information processing", and his feeding model, like the control system of Payne and Dugdale (1977), does not use a set point reference system.

The existence (or not) of a set point is of fundamental importance in our understanding of human obesity, since if it exists it is possible that obesity is a condition in which the control system is working normally, but the set point for body fat is too high. I have argued against this idea (Garrow, 1974b) and will do so again in Chapter 6, but will here review data relevant to human food intake to see if a set point theory is tenable.

The short-term control of food intake in man is so erratic that it is difficult to detect *any* sort of regulation from day to day, still less any set point. In the military cadets studied over a period of 14 days by Edholm et al. (1955) energy intake and expenditure varied from day to day by a factor of two, and there was no significant correlation between the two. Even when the average intake and expenditure of each of the 12 cadets is compared over the whole 14-day study the correlation is insignificant (Garrow, 1974b). The results of the study by Garry et al. (1955) on 19 miners and 10 clerks for 1 week also fails to show a correlation between mean intake and expenditure which is significant at the 5% level. The disguised preload experiments of Walike et al. (1969), Wooley et al. (1972) and Pudel and Oetting (1977) demonstrate that both fat and lean subjects are very fallible in assessing their own energy intake and making the appropriate adjustments to the size of the following meal. The observations of

Ashworth et al. (1962) that an intragastric load of 2000 kcal (8.4 MJ) nightly for 36 nights had no detectable effect on the voluntary daily food consumption of normal volunteers may seem incredible, but a careful review of the evidence shows that short-term regulation of intake in man is indeed feeble (Garrow, 1974b).

Long-term control of intake must be quite good, since body weight in most people is fairly stable. Hervey (1969) and Bray (1976) use this as evidence of the precision of the control system, but the argument is not quite fair. Thus Bray (1976) says that the Ten State Nutrition Survey showed that the weight of white males "remained within 2 kg of the weight at age 30 until after age 60", but this is a variant of the "constancy fallacy" (see Section 2.6.1). In fact the Framingham study (Gordon and Kannel, 1973) shows that it is very rare indeed for a white male to remain within 2 kg of his weight at age 30 until after age 60; on average they will vary by about 10 kg. Even Fox (1973), who has a very stable weight, has from time to time wandered about 4 kg from his normal weight of 74 kg.

This is important if we are trying to understand the nature of the control system: it only confuses the issue if we are told to look for a system which has a maximum error of 2 kg when really it has an average error of 10 kg, since 10 kg is a change which is obvious to the individual and his friends, and hence may prompt conscious correction, while 2 kg is not. I have made this point before (Garrow, 1974b, 1976), and it seems obvious enough, but I will try to make it again since evidently several workers in the field do not accept it. An analogy may be helpful. Probably large motor insurance companies can predict accurately how much they will pay out each year on accident claims: let us suppose it is £ 20 per insured car per year. It certainly would not help a researcher trying to find out the cause of road traffic accidents if he started from the premise that every motorist had some set point of accident proneness which resulted in him having £ 20 of accident damage annually! Obviously this is not so, and among 10 motorists 9 may have no claim and the tenth claims for £ 200 during the year under consideration.

The facts concerning the stability of body weight are well known, but tend to be obscured by statements of the "constancy fallacy" type, and rather loose qualitative statements. Thus Goodner and

Ogilvie (1974) comment on "the remarkable stability of body weight" in a diabetic population who visited their clinic in Seattle at least 5 times between 1965 and 1970. Most of their 174 cases made between 5 and 10 visits, the average duration of followup was about 2 years, and a computer analysis showed that among the patients treated with insulin the slope of body weight tended to be an increase of 0.31 kg/year, while among the 133 cases treated with diet and oral agents the trend of body weight was a decrease of 0.6 kg/year. The average weight among the 41 patients on insulin was 74 kg, and the average coefficient of variation about their regression line was 3.7%. Those on oral agents had an average weight of 77 kg with a coefficient of variation of 4.6%. Is this "remarkable stability of body weight"? It is a matter of opinion, but I am not impressed. The typical patient who attended 5 times in 2 years probably had two visits fairly close together at first, with perhaps 6-month follow-up visits. On average his weight would change by about 1 kg over the 2-year period, so if he was 77 kg at the first and second visit and 76 at the last visit, what would his weight have to be on the third and fourth visit to achieve an average coefficient of variation of 4.6%? If he weighed 82 kg at his third visit and 72 kg at the fourth visit this would satisfy the requirement of having an average decrease of about 1 kg in 2 years with a coefficient of variation of 4.6%. This is considering the *average* coefficient of variation: among the patients on oral agents the standard deviation of the coefficient of variation was 7.8 on a mean of 4.6! Thus there must have been some very large fluctuations indeed in body weight in some individuals, yet the authors are impressed that "In the majority of our patients it was found that body weight was remarkably stable and not influenced by changes in therapy or severity of the metabolic abnormality."

I will return to the control of body weight and fat stores in Chapter 6: for the present it is enough to note that if there is a set point in the regulation of the body weight of an individual then it is a point from which most people stray by 5 kg or so above or below. It is contrary to the evidence to think of individuals running along predetermined tracks of body weight which typically increase by about 3 kg between age 25 and 35 years, about 2 kg between 35 and 45 years and about 1 kg between 45 and 55 years, although those are the figures which apply to averages of population groups which take out life insurance (Donald, 1973). It would be more in harmony with actual observation to think of the system which controls body weight *in an individual* having the same characteristics as that which is sometimes used to control guard dogs who have to patrol the boundary of a property: they are tethered to a ring which is free to slide along a rail parallel to the fence. The characteristics of the rail determines the *average* position of populations of such guard dogs, but at any one time the position of the guard dog is limited by the length of the tether. To apply this analogy to human body weight the long-term stability noted by Bray (1976) represents the 2-kg shift in the position of the rail as we age from 30 to 60 years, but the 10-kg short-term fluctuations noted in the Framingham study, and in long stay prisoners, and in populations in mining or rural districts of Wales (Garrow, 1974b) represents the length of the tether. It seems more likely to yield a better understanding of the failure of regulation which results in obesity if we seek the nature of the tether, rather than plotting the layout of the rail.

4.4.6. *How is body weight sensed in man?*

For many years scientists have debated how the control system (whatever it may be) knows the magnitude of the body stores which it is regulating. Even the most profound sceptic can hardly doubt that it is necessary for any conceivable control system to know either the amount, or the change in the amount, or the variable which it is controlling. Experiments involving cross-circulation in parabiotic rats show that there are signals which inform one rat about the state of energy stores of its partner, and these signals may well occur in man also. However, if you ask any non-scientist how he knows if his weight is increasing or decreasing he will tell you (if you can persuade him that the question is not some sort of hoax) that he relies on his bathroom scales or the fit of his clothes. This point is so obvious that it tends to be overlooked.

In the short-term regulation man does not match energy intake to energy deficit or excess (Garry et al., 1955; Edholm et al., 1955, 1970; Walike et al., 1969; Wooley et al., 1972; Garrow, 1974b; Pudel and Oetting, 1977). Performance over a longer period with food of varying energy density has been investigated by Wooley (1971). He gave inmates in the Indiana Reformatory unlimited quantities of a liquid food which provided either 1.47 kcal (6.14 kJ)/ml or 0.81 kcal (3.39 kJ)/ml. There was a 5-day run-in period, and then obese and normal subjects were given either the high or low energy density food for 5 days, then crossed to the other recipe. Texture, appearance and flavour were held constant, so the test was to see if these subjects adjusted their intake to consume a constant amount of energy as rats would do (Adolph, 1947). Wooley (1971) found partial compensation for the change in energy density in both obese and normal weight subjects, but intake was still higher on the high energy density food. Ashworth (1974) and Fomon et al. (1971) have found similar results with children. Durrant et al. (1977) adopted a different design and offered obese subjects a constant amount of energy (1.55 MJ or 2.90 MJ) but with food at high or low energy density at each energy level. The purpose was to see if the subjects rated the food more satisfying when it was diluted with acaloric fluid, but a paired sequential design failed to show any significant effect. A further trial shows that this experimental design does produce a significant difference in estimated intake if there is in fact a difference in the energy value of the food offered (Durrant and Mann, 1977).

Spiegel (1973), who seems unaware of the publication by Wooley (1971), sought answers to the questions: Does man regulate his caloric intake? Is regulation accomplished by changes in meal size or meal frequency or both? What is the precision of regulation? Her subjects were normal weight students or employees at the University of Pennsylvania, the food was chocolate flavoured drink with energy densities ranging from 0.25 to 1.8 kcal/ml with gelatin as a thickener in the low energy density formulae. (The contribution of the gelatin to the energy content of the formula seems to have been ignored.) The results showed that there was no adjustment from meal to meal for changes in energy density. When the experiment was continued for 10–21 days with a diet providing either 0.5 or 1.0 kcal/ml the results vary between subjects. There were 15 subjects in the study, but of these the results of 3 are not given in detail and are classified as "questionable": their observed weight change did not tally well with calculated energy intake, and the author evidently believes that they may have broken the arrangement to eat only the liquid chocolate food provided for this experiment. Among the remaining 12, half are classified as "non-regulators", since they made no compensation for dilution of the food by eating more of it. During the period on half-strength food their energy intake was 40, 44, 50, 50, 51 and 59% of that on full-strength food. More interesting are the "regulators", who after dilution took 77, 80, 87, 88, 89 and 103% of the energy compared with the full-strength food, and each one of these 6 regulators increased both the size of meals and the average number of meals per day. The results of subject W.S. who achieved 103% adjustment are shown in detail. He took on average 3086 ml (and hence 3086 kcal) of the full-strength food during the first week of the experiment, ranging from about 2300 on the first Monday to about 3900 on the Saturday. After the substitution of diluted food on the Monday of the second week he took about 3500 ml which provided only 1750 kcal. The next day he took about 4100 ml, and thereafter over 6000 ml daily for the next 7 days, thus achieving overall 103% compensation for the dilution during the 9-day period. When on the Wednesday of the third week he was switched back to the full-strength food he took only 3200 ml, and for the next 4 days varied between 2900 and 4800 ml and kcal. These results, like those of Hashim and Van Itallie (1965) and Campbell et al. (1971), show that over a week or so some people can adjust their intake of liquid food to compensate for a change of energy density, but not everyone can, and those that do so take time to adjust and are not very accurate. Cowgill (1928) obtained similar results with dogs.

The experiments of Hashim and Van Itallie (1965), Campbell et al. (1971), Wooley (1971) and Spiegel (1973) were carefully designed so that the subjects were as far as possible deprived of external cues concerning their intake: they could not judge accurately how much they were taking of the food which was monotonous and not their normal diet, and every effort was made to eliminate changes in texture or flavour which would signal a change in energy density. Under these experimental circumstances most people do not regulate well, but these are not the circumstances in which most people are required to regulate energy intake. In my judgement the interesting question is: "Why, in real life, do most people maintain a fairly steady weight over many years, but with short-term oscillations of about 10 kg?" It is paradoxical that long-term regulation is accurate when short-term regulation is so poor. To some extent the paradox can be resolved by considering the adaptations in energy expenditure which occur with long-term overfeeding or underfeeding: these are discussed in Chapter 5. However, it is also possible that some internal monitor of the energy stores of the body has what in engineering is termed backlash: thus if the direction of drive of a geartrain is reversed the driven wheel does not start to move until the driver has taken up all the looseness in the system and starts to transmit power in the new direction. It might be that intake is regulated by something like the size of fat cells, as Faust et al. (1977) have recently suggested, and that the 10 kg oscillations in body weight which are observed in man indicate the change in fat cell size which is necessary to switch the signal from "eat more" to "eat less" or vice versa.

To test hypotheses of this type I started an experiment in April 1973 of which Fig. 4.1 summarises the results (Garrow and Stalley, 1975). At that time it seemed that my preferred weight was around 75 kg, since I had remained at about that weight without conscious effort for many years. In order to establish a baseline I continued to weigh myself for 100 days, and then overate as much as possible to drive my weight upwards. The main purpose of this part of the experiment was to see if it was possible to demonstrate a change in fat cell number in adults during overfeeding or underfeeding, but the result was inconclusive (Ashwell and Garrow, 1973). Having by August 1974 achieved a weight of about 81 kg the second set of fat biopsies were taken, I stopped deliberately overeating, and my weight began to decrease rapidly.

I was impressed by this manifestation of weight homeostasis and assumed that some control system would now return my weight to its accustomed level around 75 kg. To ensure that this was not achieved by conscious control I was weighed by a colleague and took care not to obtain external clues to my weight change. As soon as I ceased to know my weight the decrease stopped, so throughout the months of September and October 1973 it hovered between 79 and 80 kg. By November I was informed that the attempt to show spon-

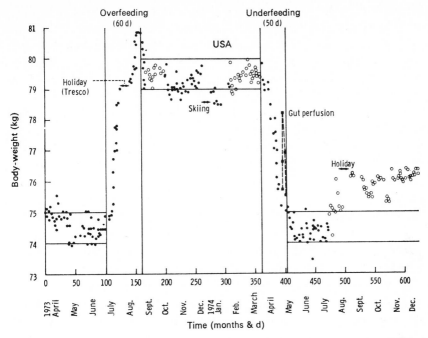

Fig. 4.1. Body weight of the author between April 1973 and December 1974. In July and August 1973 food intake was increased, and in April and May 1974 it was deliberately decreased. Otherwise no conscious effort was made to control food intake. Weights shown by filled circles were known to the subject, those shown by open circles were "blind".

taneous reversion of weight to the 75 kg "normal" had failed, so it now seemed appropriate to test the hypothesis that *knowing* my weight, without actually trying to change it, would be enough to restore it to "normal". As can be seen from Fig. 4.1 this theory was not confirmed: over Christmas 1973 there was a modest decrease to about 78.5 kg following a skiing holiday with indifferent catering facilities, but a visit to the United States followed by a period of "blind" weighing in my laboratory left me in April 1974, exactly one year after the start of the experiment, still 5 kg above what I thought was my "normal" weight.

The next step was evidently to see if it was *possible* to reduce my weight to normal. Since I am in the habit of telling obese patients that it is perfectly possible to reduce weight by 1 lb/week by dietary restriction I took my own advice and was gratified to find that it was true, although not as easy as I had expected. Thus between May and July 1974 my weight was again "normal". In order to demonstrate that this was spontaneous and not due to conscious control, I was weighed "blind" for the rest of the year and was slightly surprised to find that during the period of 4 months from August to December my weight had drifted up to about 76 kg. The results of this rather trivial experiment were communicated to the Nutrition Society (Garrow and Stalley, 1975), and among the comments at the meeting was one from Dr. Otto Edholm, a veteran investigator of energy balance in man. He said he was confident (for reasons not stated) that had the original change in body weight been downward rather than upward it would have spontaneously reverted to "normal" levels. At the time there seemed little need to confirm or refute this prediction, but for reasons connected with measurement of muscle protein turnover rate measurement (Halliday and McKeran, 1975) it became necessary for someone to lose weight rapidly in order to investigate the effect on protein turnover and metabolic rate. Thus I became involved with a continuation of the experiment to answer Edholm's point, the results of which are shown in Fig. 4.2. This experiment began in April 1975, and since a rapid weight loss was required for other reasons a minimum rate of loss of 1 kg/week was included in the protocol: in fact the target loss of 7 kg was achieved in 31 days. Thereafter food intake was not consciously controlled and weight was recorded "blind" to see if Edholm's prediction was upheld. This part of the experiment was communicated to the Nutrition Society by Garrow and Stalley (1977).

The plan was that I would avoid external clues to my weight as far as possible, and the experiment would terminate when my weight had reached a stable level for 3 months. However, this design was frustrated by events, since by February 1976 I was unable to ignore the fact that my clothes were unusually tight, so I could not maintain the "blind" condition which was required. By March 1976 there seemed little to be gained by continuing, so I was shown the weight record, and in a leisurely fashion reduced my weight by eating a bit less until my clothes fitted reasonably well.

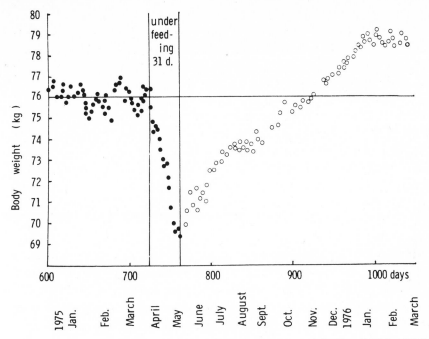

Fig. 4.2. Weight chart of the subject studied by Garrow and Stalley (1975, 1977). ●, weight known to the subject; ○, weight not known.

It is a fair criticism that this is a saga of poorly conceived hypotheses and badly controlled experimental conditions, but it may still yield information about the control of food intake in man which could not be obtained in shorter experiments, however well planned they might be. In interpreting these results it is first necessary to establish what my "normal" weight is. In April 1973 it seemed to be about 75 kg, but it is noticeable that weights around this value in Figs. 4.1 and 4.2 are mostly marked by filled circles: in other words this is a weight I tend to be when I know my weight, but the "blind" weights show no tendency to keep to this value. It might be argued that my "normal" weight is around 79 kg, since "blind" weights tend to converge on this value, but I feel sure that they stopped there in February 1976 (Fig. 4.2) because my clothes were tight. It is interesting, but fruitless, to speculate what would have happened if I habitually wore the loose robes associated with Middle Eastern countries. If I spend my time about 4 kg below my "normal" weight then I am a "restrained eater" in the nomenclature of Herman and Mack (1975), and perhaps even "latent obese" in the classification of Pudel and Oetting (1977), but if so I am not aware of it.

4.4.7. S.E.O.O.A.H. proposal

In the last 6 years there have been at least 8 major international conferences concerned with the regulation of energy balance and obesity in man: on energy balance in Paris (1971) and Lausanne (1974), Fogarty meetings in Washington on obesity (1973 and 1977), International Congresses on obesity in London (1974) and Washington (1977), on hunger in Los Angeles (1975) and on appetite in Berlin (1975), as well as many other meetings of physiologists and behavioural scientists seeking to know what controls eating and drinking. It is fair to say that the proceedings of the conferences listed above provide much more information about the regulation of food intake in rats, or about short-term regulation in man, than they do about long-term regulation in man.

The main thrust of this chapter is that man is not a rat (Edholm, 1973), and that in man short-term regulation gives us little insight into the mechanism of long-term regulation. Of course long-term regulation in man is very difficult and tedious to study, as Figs. 4.1 and 4.2 illustrate. However, the experts who have contributed to the conferences listed above constitute a body of over 100 dedicated scientists, and I believe that our knowledge in this field would advance quite quickly if they (or any reader of this book) joined S.E.O.O.A.H.

There is no membership fee, you do not require a seconder, there are no meetings, for the purpose of the Society for Enquiry into One's Own Alimentary Habits is that members who during working hours observe the effect of hypothalamic lesions on the weight of rats (or similar projects) should also record their own body weight and seek to record the factors which influence it. There is a distinguished tradition of enquiry along these lines: the founding fathers of S.E.O.O.A.H. are such men as Neumann (1902) and Gulick (1922), so professional scientists need not be ashamed to join in. It is not proposed that members should undergo great trials of overfeeding or deprivation, since we need to know more about the trivial things which deflect energy balance one way or the other in normal people, and still more we need to know what stops weight drifting upwards or downwards when the balance is upset. Each individual can only effectively study himself, but it is rare for this much to appear in scientific publications, and usually it is revealed accidentally. For example the paper by Forbes and Reina (1970) is intended to show (and does show) that lean body mass is remarkably stable in any one individual and tends to decline with age. Fig. 4.3 is taken from that paper and shows body weight and lean body mass in two subjects, A.B. and E.A., over a long period of time. (I can think of two scientists with similar initials who have been concerned with measurement of body composition over the relevant period.) The tantalising feature of the diagram is the total body weight curve. Why did A.B. show those sharp decreases in weight at age 36, 54, 61 and 64, and why did it increase in between? Was it part of some experimental protocol, or was it just drift in the control system which from time to time he consciously corrected? E.A. shows more gradual fluctuations, but still with an amplitude of about 10 kg. Were they intentional, and if not, does he know why they occurred?

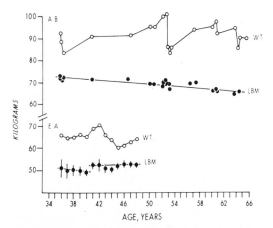

Fig. 4.3. Longitudinal study of body weight and lean body mass of two subjects. (Reprinted from Forbes and Reina (1970) with permission.)

During the preparation of this book I have spent many hours reading and writing between 23.00 and 06.00 h, when normally I am asleep. To work efficiently in the small hours I take coffee and biscuits which I would not normally take, and my weight tends to increase. Is this general experience: do the fluctuations shown by A.B. and E.A. correspond to cycles of literary activity? If rats showed these fluctuations it would be a legitimate cause for enquiry, but the text of Forbes and Reina (1970) tells us nothing about the fluctuations of fat content in these two subjects, but notes that the increase in lean body mass in subject E.A. at age 41 may be "a reported increase in physical activity at that time."

4.5. Summary: the control of food intake in man

The dual centre hypothesis for the control of food intake has recently been revised: the lateral hypothalamic nucleus is concerned with arousal rather than hunger, and the loss of satiety with ventromedial lesions in the rat is attributable to damage to fibres close to the ventromedial nucleus rather than to destruction of a satiety centre in the nucleus itself. Signals from many sources converge on the hypothalamus: their origin and routes are incompletely understood, but they are both neural and hormonal and involve the gut and liver as well as the cerebral cortex.

In man control of food intake is very complex, and the primitive hypothalamic reflexes are buried under so many layers of conditioning, cognitive and social factors that they are barely discernible. In the short term the physiological control of food intake is very poor, and under laboratory test conditions he is easily mislead by false cognitive clues. Body weight in man is not constant within 2 kg, as has been stated, but usually fluctuates about 10 kg during the adult life-span.

The factors determining these short-term (i.e. year to year) oscillations are unknown, and virtually uninvestigated except on an anecdotal basis. It would be helpful if workers in the field at least recorded their own body weight, as well as that of their experimental animals. Man's brain is so large, and its activity so obtrusive, that it is unlikely that any laboratory animal will serve as a satisfactory model for the long-term control of food intake in man. The solution recommended was well put by Alexander Pope over 200 years ago:

> Know then thyself, presume not God to scan,
> The proper study of mankind is man.

CHAPTER 5

Factors affecting energy output

The energy cost of resting metabolism, like the normal pressure of the atmosphere or the gravitational field of the earth, is always with us and is consistently underestimated. If, in hurricane winds or a wildly swerving car, we are buffetted about by a change in the magnitude or direction of these forces of pressure or acceleration, it is a frightening and impressive experience, but on calm reflection it can be seen that the magnitude of the forces involved are very small compared with the static pressure which is so familiar that we forget it.

It is easy, therefore, to understand why the lay public expect their total energy expenditure to be closely related to the level of physical activity and think that while at rest they are using no energy. It is less easy to understand why a distinguished physiologist like Buskirk (1974) should say "Cold exposure and exercise are the only significant factors leading to increased energy expenditure under our usual conditions of life style." Buskirk et al. (1960) showed that men clad only in shorts and exposed to an air temperature of 50°F for 3–6 h increased their metabolic rate by about 50%, but these circumstances are no part of most peoples' usual conditions of life style. Similarly, in extreme conditions energy expenditure can be greatly increased by physical activity: champion skiers competing in 24 h cross-country events may use 7000 kcal (29 MJ) in a day, but again this is probably not their usual life style, and it is unlikely that they could repeat the performance the next day.

A more realistic estimate of the extra energy expenditure which can be achieved by physical activity within the limits of "usual conditions of life style" can be obtained from the experience of Gwinup (1975). He attempted to treat 34 obese patients (29 women and 5 men) by encouraging them to walk vigorously for at least 30 min/day for at least a year. Only 11 patients (all women) achieved this target.

He calculates the energy expenditure of walking at 300 kcal/h, and assumes that those few patients who walked 2 h a day should have expended 600 kcal more than those who did not walk, and was disappointed that the observed rate of weight loss was not about 1 kg/week as he hoped, but "rarely exceeded 0.5 lb (0.23 kg) weekly and was usually less." He concludes that the patients must have eaten more, to explain their poor rate of weight loss. This is a common fallacy among advocates of physical exercise to promote weight loss: they assume the gross cost of the exercise is also the net cost, which is plainly nonsense. If the women had not been walking and expending (say) 5 kcal/min, they would have been doing something else for those 2 h, probably with a cost of about 2 kcal/min. Thus the cost of 120 min of vigorous walking is not $120 \times 5 = 600$ kcal, but $120 \times (5 - 2) = 360$ kcal.

Buskirk (1974) observes "If daily energy expenditure exceeds 4000 kcal/day, obesity is seldom seen." No reference is given for this statement, which would be difficult to disprove. Anyone who uses 4000 kcal/day probably expends about 3000 of them during his 16 waking hours, which gives an average rate of energy expenditure during the day of over 3 kcal/min throughout the 16 h. It is at least a tenable explanation of Buskirk's observation (if it is true) that few obese people could sustain this rate of working. Certainly intermittent

TABLE 5.1

FACTORS KNOWN TO AFFECT ENERGY EXPENDITURE IN MAN

	Inevitable	Variable
Resting metabolism	Age Sex (? genes)	Diet Lean body mass Temperature Hormones Drugs (poisons) (?) Stress
Muscular work		Level of activity Body weight Training and clothing (?) Diet

strenuous exercise is no protection against obesity, as can be seen from the study of Nishizawa et al. (1976) on the sumo wrestlers of Japan.

The factors which are known to affect energy expenditure in man are set out in Table 5.1. In my assessment the factors which are shown to act on resting metabolic rate are at least as important quantitatively as those concerned with physical activity.

5.1. Resting metabolic rate

The difference between resting metabolic rate (RMR) and basal metabolic rate (BMR) is somewhat academic. The earliest clinical application of indirect calorimetry was to investigate thyroid disease, and at the Mayo Clinic in the 1920s the group under Boothby performed a vast number of determinations of what they termed "basal metabolic rate". The BMR is defined as the energy output of an individual under standardised resting conditions: bodily and mentally at rest, 12—18 h after a meal, and in a neutral thermal environment. Strictly speaking it is also necessary to define the conditions with respect to circadian rhythms, which persist throughout the day, however rigorously the environment may be controlled (Aschoff and Pohl, 1970). Thus oxygen consumption falls in the early hours of the morning, whether or not the subject is asleep. In women this circadian rhythm persists, but the oxygen uptake is consistently lower postmenstrually than it is premenstrually. Cyclical variations in body temperature are well known, and in the rabbit these may persist even after ovariectomy (Kihlström and Lundberg, 1971). There are similar circadian rhythms in human urinary amino acid excretion (Tewksbury and Lohrenz, 1970) and in the plasma-free amino acids (Feigin et al., 1971) which persist regardless of diet or exercise.

In practice it is far more difficult to achieve the conditions of "basal metabolism" than it is to define them. Given a suitably cooperative subject it is easy to arrange that he has the measurement done in a neutral thermal environment 12—18 h after a meal; the problems arise when you try to measure his oxygen consumption under conditions of mental and physical rest. For indirect calorimetry it is essential that all the expired gases are collected: if any is lost the measurement is invalid. Therefore the subject must wear some form of mask or mouthpiece which seals perfectly to his face, and only well-trained subjects can approximate to mental and physical rest in these circumstances. Even quite minor disturbances in the room cause a change of 10% in the oxygen uptake of a trained subject at rest. The effects of disturbance on "basal" metabolism have been discussed in Section 3.2.6 and are illustrated in Fig. 3.2.

It is understandable that the early investigators should have chosen to measure "basal" metabolic rate in order to obtain readings which were as reproducible as possible, but it is evident that even so they had difficulty in obtaining technically satisfactory measurements. Boothby and Sandiford (1929) report that at the Mayo Clinic up to December 1926 measurements of BMR had been performed on more than 60,000 individuals, but when they came to report their normal values they used only "6888 subjects (1822 male and 5066 female), who on careful physical examination revealed no abnormality which would influence their rate of heat production" and who also had technically satisfactory recordings. The later definitive "standard for basal metabolism, with a nomogram for clinical application" (Boothby et al., 1936) was based on an even more selected sample of the total available measurements. One of the tenets of the Mayo Clinic, which has been rather uncritically accepted up to the present day, is that it is appropriate to express basal metabolism in relation to the subjects' surface area. This quaint idea has an interesting history.

It was observed that when physiological measurements of many kinds (such as glomerular filtration rate) were made on individuals of different size, the larger individuals gave higher values. Thus, if the observer was asked if a given patient had a high or low glomerular filtration rate, he had to make some correction for body size. Simply to divide by body weight was not satisfactory, since in general, people who weigh 120 kg do not have double the glomerular filtration rate of those who weigh 60 kg. McIntosh et al. (1929) thought it reasonable to correct renal clearance rates by dividing by the weight of the kidneys, but this cannot be determined in living human subjects: however, further research revealed that kidney weight was quite well correlated with body surface area on the evidence of post-mortem data. Thus it came about that renal clearance rates were quoted relative to surface area, and, since medico-actuarial tables of the time stated that the average area of normal young men was 1.73 m², nephrologists "corrected" renal clearance measurements to a value of 1.73 m². All this was empirical and perfectly sensible within its limitations. However, the limitations were soon exceeded, and physiologists noted with delight that the basal metabolic rates of mice and elephants, and of species of intermediate size, were fairly similar when related to their surface area. The temptation to elevate this observation to the status of a Physiological Law was irresistible: it was pointed out that surface area determined rate of heat loss, and basal metabolism the rate of heat production, so it was inevitable that the two were inextricably linked.

It is clear to anyone who has given the matter thought that, in the human species at least, the BMR is not determined by the rate of heat loss. If this were so the BMR would be higher if the subject is lying spread-eagled, and thus presenting the maximum area for heat loss, than if he curled up in as small a volume as possible, but this is not so. The conditions for measurement of BMR specifically require a neutral thermal environment, so even if there were a heat loss effect (as of course there is when the range of shivering thermogenesis is reached) it would not be detected by the test.

It is astonishing, therefore, that basal metabolic rate is still often reported in relation to surface area, or, more obscurely, as a percentage of "normal" values which have themselves been derived using surface area as a parameter. It would be understandable if in practice it worked well, but it does not. The traditional Du Bois formula for calculating surface area gives an answer which is about 6.6% too low, and has a coefficient of variation of 11% (Van Graan and Wyndham, 1964). In practice body weight is as good a reference standard as calculated surface area (Durnin, 1959).

The case for abandoning the "BMR" and substituting "resting metabolism" is well made by Durnin and Passmore (1967). The 12–18-h period of fasting is inconvenient for the subject, and if the measurement of metabolic rate is made 2–4 h after a light breakfast as much is gained by making the test less trying, as is lost by abandoning the true fasting state. The problem of correction for body size remains, but, before deciding *how* to correct for body size, it is important to be clear *why* we should correct for body size. Usually we should not do so; certainly in the study of energy balance it is nonsense to measure the energy cost of every other activity in kcal/min, and that of basal metabolism in $kcal/m^2/min$. The problem of correcting for body size arises only when it is necessary to say if a given resting metabolic rate is "normal" or not, or when the metabolic rates of subjects of very different build are being compared. Durnin and Passmore (1967) give a somewhat arbitrary, but very useful, table of normal values for resting oxygen consumption in adults of average build, and this is a better reference standard than tables based on "surface area", for reasons given above. When the problem arises of defining the "normal" resting metabolic rate of a grossly obese person weighing, for example, 150 kg, it is as well to recognise that there is no such thing as a normal value for an abnormal person. It may be informative to compare the observed metabolic rate of such a patient with the normal rate for a person of the same height and normal build, but anyone who gives values for the metabolic rate of obese patients as "percent normal for surface area" is not thinking about what he is doing.

5.1.1. Factors affecting resting metabolic rate

The factors which affect resting metabolic rate, and the publications on this topic, have been reviewed in some detail recently (Garrow, 1974b, 1978). It would be more appropriate to summarise the important points here and refer the interested reader to these reviews than to give a detailed analysis once more. However, when the views stated here are contrary to the conclusions of other workers in the field the reasons for dissent will be explained, so the reader can make his own judgement.

5.1.2. Age, sex, body weight and composition

Children have a higher metabolic rate than adults expressed either in relation to body weight or surface area. Indeed, it is one of the simplest illustrations of the fact that resting metabolic rate is not determined by surface area that a child of 5 years has a heat output of about $55-60\,\text{kcal/m}^2\text{/h}$, while an adult has about $35-40\,\text{kcal/m}^2\text{/h}$ at age 20 and about $30-33\,\text{kcal/m}^2\text{/h}$ at age 70. The argument that different species have a constant metabolic rate in relation to surface area cannot be taken very seriously when within our own species there is roughly a halving of metabolic rate per m^2 during our life-span. The metabolic rate of men is about 15% higher than that of women of the same body mass and shape.

The high metabolic rate of children is easily explained by the energy cost of growth (Millward et al., 1976; Spady et al., 1976). The higher metabolic rate of men than women is explained by the greater lean body mass in men (or greater fat mass in women). There is some controversy on this last point, since Bray et al. (1970) found that in massively obese patients metabolic rate was more closely related with fat mass than with measures of lean body mass. This finding is contrary to our own results and the great majority of the literature reviewed by (among others) Bray (1976). The explanation is that the measures of lean body mass used by Bray et al. (1970) were inappropriate for very obese patients. This point is discussed further in Chapter 6, Section 6.2.2.

Miller and Parsonage (1975) also found a better correlation between metabolic rate and estimates of fat mass than lean mass in 29 obese women who were particularly resistant to weight loss on a reducing diet, and it is not easy to explain their results. Of course lean mass and fat mass are themselves correlated, so even if there was no direct correlation between fat and metabolic rate there would be an association of subjects with high fat mass and high metabolic rate due to common association with lean mass. The analysis of this problem when 3 factors are each related to the other must be by stepwise regression, so the contribution of one factor to the total variance is measured, and then the effect of the second factor in explaining the remaining variance is tested. However, this procedure gives an advantage to the factor entered at the first step, as can be illustrated by the example below.

Consider the 22 women studied by Halliday et al. (1978). They weighed 90.2 kg (± 18.6), and estimates of lean body mass by total body potassium gave a value of 48.6 ± 7.3 kg, leaving 41.6 ± 13.8 kg of fat mass. When body composition was measured by total body water the estimated lean mass was 50.1 ± 8.1 kg leaving 40.1 ± 14.5 kg for fat mass. Their observed resting oxygen uptake ranged from 212 to 356 ml/min, and simple correlation of lean mass with resting metabolic rate gave a correlation coefficient of 0.844 when the potassium method was used, and 0.759 when the water method was used, both being significant at $P < 0.001$. However, the correlations with fat mass are also statistically significant: 0.623 using the potassium method and 0.593 using the water method. The question to be answered is: to what extent is the association of fat mass with metabolic rate due to their common association with lean mass? A simple correlation between these two gives $r = 0.52$. A multiple regression analysis in which lean and fat mass by water or potassium are the independent variables, and resting metabolic rate the dependent variable (i.e. the thing to be predicted) is set out in Table 5.2.

TABLE 5.2

MULTIPLE REGRESSION OF LEAN AND FAT MASS ON METABOLIC RATE IN 22 WOMEN (data of Halliday et al., 1978)

Independent variable	Sums of squares	df	F	P
LBM (potassium)	18,825	1	50	<0.001
Add fat (potassium)	1 256	1	3.8	N.S.
Residual	6 319	19		
	26,400			
Fat (potassium)	10,260	1	12.7	<0.005
Add LBM (potassium)	9 821	1	29.5	<0.001
Residual	6 319	19		
	26,400			
LBM (water)	15,200	1	27.1	<0.001
Add fat (water)	3 846	1	9.9	<0.01
Residual	7 354	19		
	26,400			
Fat (water)	9 280	1	10.8	<0.005
LBM (water)	9 766	1	25.2	<0.001
Residual	7 354	19		
	26,400			

The total variation in metabolic rate among these 22 women is represented by the total in the "sums of squares" column in Table 5.2, and this is 26,400. The factor which "explains" the greatest fraction of this variation is lean body mass as estimated from total body potassium: this contributes 18,825 to the total, and adding fat "explains" only an insignificant 1256 of the residual variation. However, it should be noted that in the second calculation in Table 5.2, where fat is entered as the first independent variable it appears to do quite well, and "explains" 10,260 of the total variation. However, when lean body mass is now added it makes a more powerful contribution to the remaining variation (shown by the higher F value) than fat did at the first stage of analysis. If water is used as the basis for estimating lean and fat tissue, the results obtained are shown in the lower part of the table. Again lean tissue makes a more significant contribution to "explaining" the variation whether it is entered before or after fat tissue, but body composition estimated from total body water measurements is less satisfactory than that estimated from potassium at "explaining" variation in metabolic rate, as can be seen from the larger residual figure (7354 for water compared with 6319 for potassium). The reasons for this will be discussed in Chapter 6.

This example has been considered in some detail to show how some investigators have reached the conclusion (in my opinion wrongly) that fat has a greater relationship to metabolic rate than lean. The point is of some importance for two reasons. First, if it were true that fat mainly determined metabolic rate the outlook would indeed be dismal for the very fat patient with an average metabolic rate, since if he lost his fat he must be condemned to a greatly reduced metabolic rate and hence a difficult task in maintaining his weight loss. However if, as I believe, lean tissue determines metabolic rate there is some point in seeking lines of treatment which will cause fat loss but relatively spare lean tissue. The second reason for belabouring the issue is that if we can accept that lean tissue determines metabolic rate there is no need to seek strange explanations for the lower metabolic rate of women than men, or old people than young people. This section is headed "Age, sex, body weight and composition", because the available evidence says that the effect of all of these factors on metabolic rate is through the common factor of lean body mass. If this simple explanation fits the observations (and I think it does) there is no merit in seeking a more complex one. As that astute monk William of Occam observed about 650 years ago "Entia non sunt multiplicanda praeter necessitatem."

5.1.3. Individual variation in metabolic rate

The nomogram of Boothby and Berkson (1933) provides a convenient method for predicting the average basal metabolic rate of a group of people matched for age, sex, weight and height (or surface area). However, the clinician is usually concerned with individuals rather than groups of people, so it is obviously important to know the probable variation of individuals from this average value. Boothby et al. (1936) addressed this problem and provided details of the number of subjects who deviated from predicted metabolic rate by various margins, which differed with age and sex of the subject. Roughly speaking, in the adult age range the coefficient of variation among measurements on subjects matched for age, sex and surface area, and who "on careful physical examination revealed no abnormality which would influence their rate of heat production", was 9%. This result has been taken to mean that "normal" people have a metabolic rate within 10% of that predicted by the Boothby and Berkson nomogram, but this is clearly untrue (unless a deviation of more than 10% is taken as evidence of abnormality, in which case the statement achieves the unassailable truth of all totally circular arguments). The probability of finding a person without any detectable endocrine abnormality whose metabolic rate is 20% different from expected is certainly not negligible, especially among those individuals who select themselves by attending hospital complaining of difficulty in maintaining body weight within normal limits. Groups of obese people may not have an average metabolic rate which differs significantly from "normal", but to argue from this observation to the conclusion that individual obese patients cannot have an abnormal metabolic rate is to fall for a variant of the "constancy fallacy" mentioned in Section 2.6.1. Investigators who study patients with varying degrees of obesity find some with normal metabolic rates and some with low metabolic rates (Martineaud and Trémolière, 1964), while those who deal with the super-obese tend to be impressed with the high metabolic rate of such patients, and hence assume that all obese patients have a high metabolic rate (Bray, 1976). It can be shown that William Campbell, the British record holder for obesity who died at the age of 22 weighing 340 kg, had probably acquired an excess store of about 1,750,000 kcal in excess fat (Garrow, 1976). This would require an average daily storage of 218 kcal, or about 7% of his probable intake. It is therefore important to recognise that individuals of the same age, sex, weight and lifestyle may have differences in metabolic rate of more than 30% (Warwick et al., 1978), so it is by no means impossible that on the same diet one person would remain thin while another, apparently similar, person would become fat.

5.1.4. Effect of underfeeding on metabolic rate

It should not be necessary to elaborate on the fact that people who are on a restricted diet show a decrease in metabolic rate which is greater than that which would be expected from tissue loss. The literature has been reviewed (Garrow, 1974b) and there is no investigator who has looked for this effect and failed to find it. Probably the first report was that of Benedict et al. (1919) in their classical study of "Human vitality and efficiency under prolonged restricted diet". Their results are illustrated in Fig. 5.1.

Benedict et al. (1919) studied healthy young volunteers who took a holiday from the experiment at Thanksgiving and at Christmas. The effect is beautifully shown in the results: during the period of restricted diet resting metabolic rate fell, after brief refeeding it rose sharply but fell equally quickly when the restriction was reimposed. These results have been confirmed in normal volunteers (Keys et al., 1950) and in obese patients (Bray, 1969a; Apfelbaum et al., 1971, 1977). Our own experience is summarised in Fig. 5.2 which shows the body weight and resting oxygen uptake of 27 women on admission to the metabolic unit at the Clinical Research Centre (open circles) and the corresponding values after 3 weeks on a diet supplying 3.4 MJ (800 kcal)/day (closed circles). The upper broken regression line shows the relationship on admission, and the lower continuous

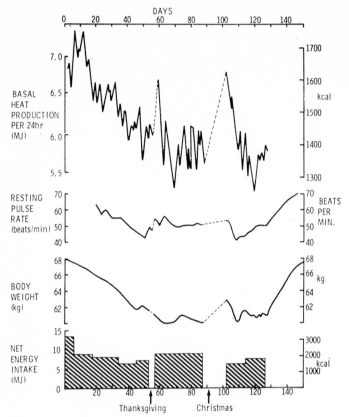

Fig. 5.1. The effect of a restricted diet on the basal metabolic rate, resting pulse rate and body weight of normal volunteers (data of Benedict et al., 1919). The experiment was interrupted for holidays at Thanksgiving and Christmas, and after 126 days the subjects ate ad libitum.

line after the 3 weeks of restricted diet.

The regression equations show that metabolic rate fell by 18 ml O_2/min *more* than would be expected for the change in weight of the group as a whole. However, the figure also illustrates the point made in 5.1.3 that there is considerable individual variation in metabolic rate among people of the same weight, and also variation in the response to the reducing diet both with respect to weight loss and change in metabolic rate.

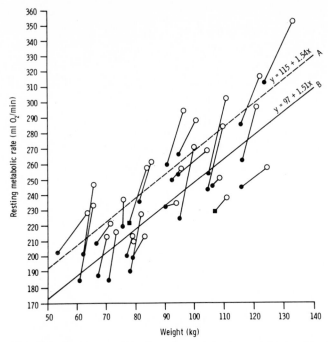

Fig. 5.2. Resting metabolic rate and body weight in 27 obese women before (open circles) and after (closed circles) 3 weeks on a diet supplying 3.4 MJ (800 kcal) daily. Data of Garrow and Warwick (1978).

5.1.5. Effect of overfeeding on metabolic rate

The climate of scientific opinion has changed considerably since an unsigned editorial in the *American Journal of Clinical Nutrition* (1970) stated: "There are no satisfactory experiments on dogs or man indicating that a luxus consumption mechanism exists." I have recently reviewed the conflicting literature on this topic (Garrow, 1978); the key publications are listed in chronological order in Table 5.3 with some simplification of the results to allow 75 years of research to be presented in a single tabulation. Only the conclusions will be stated here, since the underlying reasoning is set out elsewhere (Garrow, 1978).

TABLE 5.3

IS ENERGY EXPENDITURE INCREASED BY OVERFEEDING IN MAN?

Authors	Date	Subjects		Days overfed	Excess (Mcal)	Increased RMR?	Unexplained energy loss	Con-clusion
		Fat	Lean					
Neumann	1902	—	1	365	?100	?	yes	yes
Gulick	1922	—	1	73	51	?	yes	yes
Passmore et al.	1955	—	3	14	22	yes	NO	NO
Mann et al.	1955	—	3	20	60	?	(no) yes	yes
Ashworth et al.	1962	—	3	36	72	?	yes	yes
Passmore et al.	1963	2	—	9	10	yes	NO	NO
Miller et al.	1967	—	4	50	70	yes	(yes)	yes
Strong et al.	1967	9	7	4	6	yes	NO	NO
Sims et al.	1968	—	9	160	400	?	yes	yes
Durnin and Norgan	1969	—	4	42	70	yes	no (?)	no
Apfelbaum et al.	1971	8	—	15	23	yes	–	yes
Whipp et al.	1973	—	4	35	120	yes	–	yes
Garrow and Stalley	1975	—	1	60	80	?	yes	yes
Goldman et al.	1976	—	4	83 (fat)	72	yes	no	yes
		—	9	18 (CHO)	33	yes	no	yes
Glick et al.	1977	4	4	5	12	no	NO	NO

The question at issue is: Does overfeeding increase energy expenditure in man? It will be seen from the last column of Table 5.3 that some authors would reply yes, and others no. However, in all the studies except that of Glick et al. (1977) it was observed that resting metabolic rate was increased. The dissent concerns the "unexplained energy loss" column. Some studies, like those of Goldman et al. (1976) can account for all the excess energy fed to the subjects, but conclude that there is a general increase in energy expenditure, hence the entry "yes" in the last column. Of great interest are the 4 publications which have the entry NO in the last two columns. The factor which these studies have in common is that the total amount of excess energy fed to the subjects was less than 22 Mcal, while in all the other publications it was more than 23 Mcal. This suggests that there is a threshold of overfeeding at which some sort of luxus consumption effect comes into action, but even very thorough studies like those of Glick et al. (1977) cannot detect any such effect with smaller overloads.

One may reasonably be accused of gerrymandering in drawing so fine a line between those studies which do, or do not, show luxus consumption, but the distinction here is not so unprincipled as that attributed to Governor Gerry. Some independent support comes from the study by Mann et al. (1955) which was mainly concerned with the effects of exercise on blood lipids during overfeeding, but during the part of the experiment abstracted in Table 5.3 the 3 subjects stopped exercising but continued to eat an excess of 3000 kcal (12 MJ) daily for the next 20 days. During the first 10 days they gained 4.7 kg, which could easily account for the excess intake, but for the next 10 days they gained only 1.3 kg, so in these subjects their response to overfeeding evidently changed as the excess mounted above some threshold of about 20 Mcal. Teleologically it is plausible that there should be a mechanism for burning off large excesses of intake which would not be triggered by a few large meals. However, it must be admitted that the mechanism of dietary induced thermogenesis is still obscure.

5.1.6. Effects of temperature on metabolic rate

It is well known that severe exposure to either heat or cold will increase metabolic rate. In subjects with fever, or who are artificially heated, metabolic rate increases by about 12% for each °C rise in deep body temperature. It has been suggested that commercially available "slimming garments" made of plastic may impair heat loss by sweating and hence increase body temperature and energy loss, but this is untrue. It is very difficult, and very unpleasant, to cause a significant increase in body temperature in this way, and the associated vasodilatation causes disabling postural hypotension.

The response to cold is well documented and also unpleasant. Buskirk et al. (1960, 1963a), Quaade (1963), Wyndham et al. (1968) and Rochelle and Horvath (1969) have all exposed nearly naked subjects to temperatures of 10°C or less. The subjects showed fortitude and an increase in metabolic rate, which was somewhat smaller in obese subjects. This is of interest, since in genetically obese mice there is a failure to respond to cold stress from an early age (Trayhurn et al., 1977) and this lack of cold-induced thermogenesis may be part of the cause of their obesity. However, it is not clear if cold-induced thermogenesis plays any important role in energy balance in real life. Jéquier et al. (1974) studied normal, moderately obese and obese women on exposure to 20°C for 120 min, and although they demonstrated differences in insulation between obese and normal women there was little difference in thermogenesis. A cold stress of 20°C is probably as great as most people would tolerate willingly, so differences in response between lean and fat subjects at 15°C, although academically interesting, are of doubtful practical importance. Fanger (1972) tested subjects seated in light clothing for 3 h at various environmental temperatures, and at the end of the test the subjects rated the conditions on a 7-point scale: −3 for much too cold, 0 for comfortable, and +3 for much too hot. The results are shown in Fig. 5.3. At 25°C there were 6% of subjects dissatisfied, half of them because it was too hot and the other half because it was too cold. As the test temperature went down the proportion complaining of cold increased to 78% at 20°C. When it was raised 79% complained that it was too hot at 32°C. When the subjects were analysed by weight-for-height there was no significant difference in the preference of the fatter subjects compared with the thinner ones.

Despite the suggestion by Buskirk (1974) that "cold exposure and

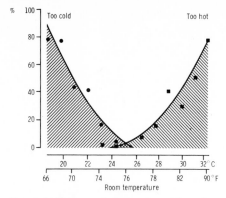

Fig. 5.3. Range of thermal comfort for subjects seated in light clothing for 3 h. Data of Fanger (1972).

exercise are the only significant factors leading to increased energy expenditure under our usual life style", we can probably delete cold exposure from this short list of possibilities, since if people are given the chance they do not expose themselves to cold severe enough to induce a metabolic response. Indeed it was Buskirk et al. (1957) who studied soldiers at military bases with ambient temperatures ranging from −25°C at Fort Churchill, Canada, to 34°C at Yuma, Ariz., and found no significant relationship between resting metabolism and climate.

5.1.7. "Specific dynamic action" or dietary thermogenesis

One or 2 h after a meal there is an increase in metabolic rate which is about 40% above basal at peak. Over the next 2 or 3 h, provided that the subject remains completely at rest, metabolic rate returns to somewhere near the basal value. The total increase over basal metabolism for 6 h after a meal supplying 1000 kcal (4.2 MJ) is about 10%. It was taught since the days of Rubner that protein had a "specific dynamic action" not possessed by carbohydrate or fat, and very careful measurements on animals support this (Blaxter, 1976), but in man our efforts to find experimental support for the suggestion by

96

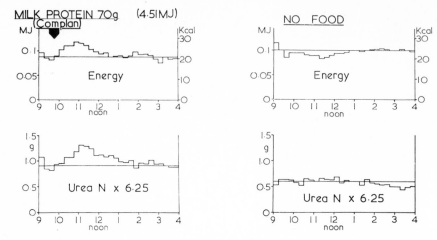

Fig. 5.4. The effect on metabolic rate, and on urea excretion, of an intragastric meal of "Complan" in a normal resting subject. The meal provided 1080 kcal (4.51 MJ) and 70 g milk protein. Energy expenditure and urea excretion are average rates for 28 consecutive periods of 15 min each (data of Garrow and Hawes, 1972).

Fig. 5.5. Metabolic rate and urea excretion in the same subject as in Fig. 5.4, who was given acaloric fluids.

Krebs (1964) that this reflected energy losses during urea production did not support this view. The results of giving meals which increased urea production (like milk protein or gelatin) or decreased it (like glucose) are shown in Figs. 5.4–5.7. It is evident that there is no association between the increase in metabolic rate after the meal and the amount of urea produced.

The thermic effect of a meal is small, and difficult to measure accurately, since for each subject it is necessary to make a prolonged measurement of metabolic rate after a meal (see Fig. 5.4) and compare this with the result which would have been obtained without the meal (see Fig. 5.5). This simple precaution of doing a control experiment without food is often omitted, but without it the thermic effect of a meal cannot be assessed. Frequently the meal is given in the morning after "baseline" measurements have been made, and it is

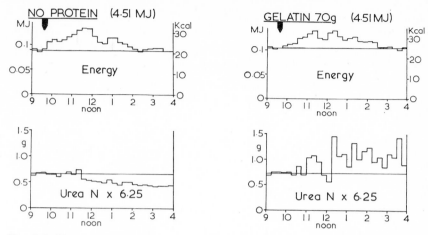

Fig. 5.6. The same experiment as in Fig. 5.4 with glucose substituted isocalorically for the milk protein.

Fig. 5.7. The same experiment as in Fig. 5.4 with gelatin substituted isocalorically for the milk protein.

tacitly assumed that had the meal not been given the metabolic rate would have remained at the baseline level. There is no reason to believe this, since the diurnal cycle in energy expenditure rises during the morning and early afternoon (Aschoff and Pohl, 1970). It is noteworthy that in the control subjects studied by Kaplan and Leveille (1976) their metabolic rate was still far above baseline 5 h after a meal providing 823 kcal, and all this increase is attributed to the meal! It might have been prudent for them to perform a control experiment, since Bradfield and Jourdan (1973) were able to show in their subjects an increase of 64% in basal metabolism in subjects who were given *no* food. It is, in fact, quite difficult to achieve the steady baseline shown in Fig. 5.5.

In view of these technical difficulties there is little reliable evidence about the relative magnitude of the thermic effect of a given meal on lean and obese subjects. The study by Pittet et al. (1976) is technically excellent and shows that in the 150 min after an oral dose of 50 g glucose 10 lean women increased their metabolic rate by 13.0%, while 11 obese women showed an increase of only 5.2%. The difference is highly significant ($P < 0.001$). Stordy et al. (1977) also report a greater thermic effect in anorectic patients than controls after 100 g glucose orally. The significance of these findings is not clear.

The thermic response to food and to cold seem to be independent. Buskirk et al. (1960) and Rochelle and Horvath (1969) tested both stimuli separately and together and found no significant interaction.

5.1.8. The effect of stress on resting metabolic rate

Stress is difficult to define, but it is generally agreed that stressful situations are tiring, and patients often imply that since they find their employment stressful it must be associated with high energy expenditure. It is true that disturbance of a resting subject causes an increase in metabolic rate transiently, as can be seen in Fig. 3.2. Certainly stress can increase heart rate (Moss and Wynar, 1970), release adrenalin and hence increase lipolysis and the concentration of free tryptophan (Gentil et al., 1977) and affect secretion of antidiuretic hormone (De Wardener, 1967). Trémolière et al. (1973) report values for resting oxygen uptake which are 25% higher when a mouthpiece is used than when measurements are made on the same subject in a respiration chamber, and they ascribe this large difference to the "vigilance" associated with wearing a rather uncomfortable mouthpiece. However, Benedict and Benedict (1933) were unable to detect any measurable effect of mental work on oxygen consumption.

It is very difficult to design an experiment in which the effect of psychological stress is not confused with the increase in muscular tension and fidgeting which stress induces. However, if a volunteer is subjected to psychological stress the increase in metabolic rate is very small even when there are large changes in heart rate, and it seems likely that stress or anxiety has no measurable effect on metabolic rate (Landis, 1925).

5.1.9. Drugs and hormones affecting metabolic rate

Dinitrophenol, salicylates and caffeine all cause an increase in metabolic rate, but probably not to an extent which would significantly affect energy balance in man, since the effect is small unless toxic doses are given.

Among the hormones thyroid derivatives are most potent in affecting metabolic rate. Epinephrine increases metabolic rate transiently with small doses, but depresses it in large doses. Growth hormone at a dose of 8 mg daily increased the rate of oxygen uptake by 10% in obese patients (Bray, 1969b). Glucagon increases oxygen uptake in rats (Davidson et al., 1960). However, these effects are not so far of practical importance, while thyroid derivatives can certainly produce a sustained increase in metabolic rate and have vogues of approbation or disrepute. The use of these drugs in the treatment of obesity is discussed in Section 7.3.2.

Recently there has been revived interest in the thyroid hormones, since better assays have been developed for triiodothyronine (T_3) which is more potent than the parent compound thyroxin (T_4) and has a shorter half-life of about 1 day (Nicoloff et al., 1972), and reversed T_3 (rT_3) which is also thyroxin with a different iodine atom removed, and which has no thermogenic effect. The mechanism by which the thyroid hormones affect metabolic rate is still not clear: their thermogenic effect is abolished if protein synthesis is blocked (Tata, 1964), but it is also argued that their effect is on the activity of the sodium pump, at least in liver, kidney and muscle (Edelman and Ismail-Beigi, 1974). Obviously all metabolic activity is not dependent on thyroid hormone, since in athyroid animals life and metabolism continues. However, recent work has shown most interesting associations between diet and the concentration of circulating thyroid hormones, especially T_3. During a fast of 60 h the concentration of T_4 and thyroid-stimulating hormone (TSH) do not significantly change, but in a study by Merimee and Fineberg (1976) the concentration of T_3 fell from 152 ng/100 ml to 131 ng/100 ml after 24 h and to 90 mg/100 ml at 60 h. The half-life of thyroxin is about 7 days, so it is too clumsy an instrument to regulate rapid responses to change in diet, but it seems that conversion of thyroxin to T_3, or alternatively to the inactive rT_3, in the peripheral tissues would provide a more nimble control system. The reduction in T_3 with fasting seems to be prevented with modest amounts of carbohydrate (Spaulding, 1976).

A most impressive study of the effects of total starvation for 10 days is reported by Palmblad et al. (1977). Their 12 normal volunteers showed a marked decrease in T_3 and heart rate during the period of starvation, there was a small decrease in T_4 and TSH and an increase in rT_3. All this fits in well with the concept of the output of thyroxin and T_3 from the thyroid gland being a rather coarse control system which is further modulated by conversion of T_4 to T_3 or rT_3 in the peripheral tissues. Palmblad et al. (1977) also report a very significant increase in growth hormone concentration in the serum after 3 days of starvation, which returned to control levels even though the fast was continued for 10 days. Cortisol increased somewhat throughout the fast, and urine adrenalin increased, but noradrenalin was not changed. The meaning of all these changes is not clear, but it is obvious that in response to the severe stress of 10 days of total starvation there are complex changes in the endocrine economy, and it is very difficult to identify which effects are primary and which secondary. The prolonged starvation of anorexia nervosa is also associated with many changes in endocrine activity. Croxson and Ibbertson (1977) report T_3 concentrations of 62 ng/100 ml in 22 patients with anorexia, which is about half the value found in normal controls. Beumont et al. (1976) reported normal TSH, prolactin and response to TSH stimulation in 15 women with anorexia, but they had low levels of luteinising hormone and follicle-stimulating hormone, which increased with weight gain. Kalucy et al. (1976) compared the nocturnal hormonal profiles of obese and anorectic women, and found that compared with normal controls both obese and anorectic women had low concentrations of growth hormone and luteinising hormone, but raised concentrations of insulin. In the anorectic women prolactin and LSH were low and cortisol was raised, whereas in obese women prolactin was raised but LSH and cortisol were normal.

Bray et al. (1976c) reported a modest but significant correlation between concentrations of T_3 and body weight in 97 patients whose weight ranged from normal to about 200 kg, and showed that when lean or obese subjects overate and gained weight there was an increase in serum T_3 concentration. Premachandra and Perlstein (1976) found thyroglobulin antibodies in some obese people but not in others. If present they could be suppressed with rather large doses of T_3.

All these results can be reconciled with the view that the decrease in metabolic rate which occurs when food intake is restricted is mediated by a decrease in the peripheral conversion of T_4 to T_3, and perhaps an increase in conversion of T_4 to the inactive rT_3. The effect of the changed concentration of thyroid hormone on metabolic rate may be through the reduced activity of the sodium pump, or by reducing protein turnover, or both observed effects may be merely examples of a reduction of active transport in general through the cell membrane. Conversely, during overfeeding the opposite effects may occur with a consequent increase in metabolic rate. However, this simple view is by no means established and leaves several interesting observations unexplained. For example it does nothing to account for the dramatic but transient spike in serum growth hormone in the fasting subjects studied by Palmblad et al. (1977), nor do we know what quantitative significance to ascribe to the observed changes in catecholamines.

Other hypotheses have been advanced for connections between endocrine disorders and obesity. Prostaglandins might inhibit lipolysis and hence promote obesity (Curtis-Prior, 1975), but there is not much evidence that failure of lipolysis is a characteristic of obese people. It may be that so-called "anorectic" drugs like mazindol or fenfluramine have a peripheral action on glucose metabolism (Kirby and Turner, 1976): there is evidence for this in vitro but not in studies of metabolic rate in man.

5.2. Muscular work and energy expenditure

Other things being equal people engaged in heavy work use about 800 kcal (3.3 MJ)/day more than people in sedentary jobs. Thus in the workers in a jute mill in West Bengal studied by Mayer et al. (1956) the men who were in the most strenuous occupations, which involved handling heavy bales of jute, used about 3600 kcal daily, while sedentary clerks used about 2800 kcal/day. In a very careful study of coal miners Garry et al. (1955) found a mean energy expenditure among 19 men hewing coal with pickaxes of 3660 kcal/day, while the average for 10 clerks was 2800 kcal/day. In their excellent review on human energy expenditure Passmore and Durnin (1955) observe that a rate of energy expenditure of 5 kcal/min is "approximately the upper limit of work which can be performed without an increasing accumulation of lactic acid and without a rise in body temperature . . . It is equivalent to a daily walk of about 30 miles . . . Work at 5 kcal/min for 8 h corresponds to 2400 kcal expended at work. If we allow 500 kcal for 8 h in bed and about 1400 kcal for the 8 h spent off work the total energy expenditure for 24 h is 4300 kcal. This probably represents the upper rates of daily energy expenditure which can be maintained regularly in heavy industry."

Certainly it is possible to expend more than 5 kcal/min over short periods in athletic events, and some of the mining activities measured by Garry et al. (1955), such as hewing coal, loading it onto conveyor belts, and timbering the cuttings, cost over 7 kcal/min. However, let us consider one of the subjects studied by Garry and his colleagues who is identified in the report as Jock E. He was a 27-year-old man, height 178 cm, weight 72.5 kg. During the week beginning August 18th 1952 he worked the regulation 5-day shifts in the mine, being wound down between 5.45 and 6.00 a.m. and wound up between 1.30 and 2.00 p.m. He also worked 3 overtime shifts, to give a total of 60 h 17 min underground during the week since, as the investigators observed, "there are strong financial inducements to work such hours". This man must have been close to "the upper rates of energy expenditure which can be maintained regularly in heavy industry", and was certainly far above the workload which would now be considered acceptable, yet his daily energy expenditure for that week averaged 4090 kcal (17.1 MJ).

This study has been reviewed in some detail because the effects of muscular work on energy expenditure tend to be exaggerated. The suggestion of Tullis (1973) that obese patients should adopt "a vigorous physical activity programme" may be good advice, but to suggest that it would involve expending "at least 1200 kcal" is absurd. Jock E. the miner working 20 h of overtime at one of the most strenuous industrial jobs just about achieved this target, but it would be interesting to know if any obese patient could manage it even for a day. At the beginning of this chapter it was pointed out that Gwinup (1975) calculated that an obese patient who walked for 2 h using

300 kcal/h should have expended 600 kcal more than a similar person who had not undertaken this exercise, and this type of calculation, based on the *gross* cost of exercise, promotes euphoria among advocates of exercise. However the true *net* cost of exercise is the gross cost less the energy cost of whatever they would have done had they not been exercising. As a rough guide the net cost of exercise for most adults is about 2 kcal/min less than the gross cost, unless the exercise is taken instead of bedrest, in which case it would be fairer to subtract about 1 kcal/min from the gross cost.

If this means of calculation is used the limitations on increasing energy expenditure by exercise become apparent. Levels of activity above 5 kcal/min cannot be sustained for very long, and activity close to 2 kcal/min has very little net effect. Thus a sedentary person who wishes to increase his energy expenditure by physical activity for 2 h daily may reasonably expect to maintain a level of activity of 5 kcal/min by walking fairly briskly for that time, with a net increase in energy expenditure of about $120 \times (5 - 2)$ kcal, which is 360 kcal, not the 600 kcal calculated by Gwinup (1975) and still less the 1200 kcal hoped for by Tullis (1973).

5.2.1. Inactivity in the aetiology of obesity

Many authors state that inactivity is an important cause of obesity, and certainly the 360 kcal (1.5 MJ), which the calculation above shows might be attributable to physical activity, would be enough to make a decisive difference to energy balance if all other factors were equal. However, to show that inactivity is a major cause of obesity requires two steps: first to show that obese people are in fact less active than lean, and second, that the difference in energy expenditure associated with physical activity is of the appropriate magnitude to explain the error in energy balance. Some authors show little regard to the quantitative aspects of the problem. Thus Buskirk (1974) says "preservation of obesity has frequently been observed at the 2200—2400 kcal/day level in men and 1800—2000 kcal level in women. Caloric balance at these levels can only be retained with low levels of physical activity." There is then a reference to Buskirk et al. (1963b) which is an excellent study of energy balance in 5 women and one man "specifically designed to determine whether we could confirm the suggested existence of the so-called "hypophagic" obese state." Their results did not confirm it, but they do not provide evidence for the statement in the later review either. Fat and thin men, and active and inactive men, can all preserve caloric balance at 2400 kcal/day.

A serious attempt to make quantitative measurements of physical activity in lean and obese subjects was made by Bloom and Eidex (1967a). By means of a clock recording device they showed that 7 obese subjects spent 529 ± 50 min in bed, and of the 911 min in the day spent out of bed 335 ± 111 min were spent standing. Among 6 lean subjects 478 ± 52 min were spent in bed, and of the remaining 962 min 525 ± 105 were spent standing. In a second paper Bloom and Eidex (1967b) report that their obese subjects had an energy consumption at rest of 1.28 kcal/min, while the lean subjects at rest used 0.77 kcal/min: thus if the obese subjects had remained in bed all day they would have used 1843 kcal/day and the lean 1109 kcal/day. To sustain the argument that "inactivity is a major factor in adult obesity" it is necessary to show that during the extra 51 min spent out of bed, with the extra 190 min which the lean subjects spent standing, more energy was used than the difference of 734 kcal in the reported basal metabolism of the two sets of subjects. Certainly the time spent out of bed but sitting could not make up the difference, since the highest reported cost of sitting in the whole series is only 1.7 kcal/min. If the extra 734 kcal were expended during the standing period of 190 min this is an extra 3.86 kcal/min above the cost of sitting, which is a highly improbable estimate for the reasons given in Section 5.2. Thus using the author's own data it is difficult to explain how the lean subjects came to use *as much* energy as the obese ones and a travesty to cite this study as evidence that inactivity is a major factor in adult obesity.

Other investigators have tried to measure the level of activity of obese and lean subjects with varying degrees of success. Stefanik et al. (1959) found no difference between 14 obese and 14 non-obese boys. McCarthy (1966) found no difference in the reported level of activity in obese and non-obese Trinidadian women. Lincoln (1972) found no difference in American adults by postal questionnaire.

Greenfield and Fellner (1969) recorded the movement of obese and non-obese females in a reclining chair and found no significant difference between the two groups. Chirico and Stunkard (1960) found that pedometer readings indicated that on average 15 obese women walked 2.0 miles/day, while lean controls walked 4.9 miles/day. Another significant finding was that the obese women tended to become more inert when despondent, while the lean controls were more likely to fight back against adversity. However, when the study was repeated on 25 obese men and a similar series of matched controls the result was not so clear, since 9 of the obese men walked further than their control, but 16 of the obese men walked less far than their lean control.

Bullen et al. (1964) went to a lot of trouble to analyse 27,211 cine photograph frames of obese and lean girls at a summer camp, and to grade the level of activity caught when the picture was taken. Not surprisingly, the obese girls who were in a camp which provided "nutritional education, dietary control and a varied activity programme for overweight girls" played volleyball and tennis less actively than lean girls who were at a different camp, and presumably played these games because they wanted to. It is not possible to say if the obese girls were less active because they were obese, or obese because they were less active, or were just inactive and obese and sent to this camp because their parents thought it would do them good.

A recent study by Wilkinson (1977) found no significant difference between the pedometer reading on 10 obese boys aged 12 years and 10 matched non-obese controls. A similar study with girls also failed to produce a significant difference.

To summarise: it is an impossible task to show that inactivity is a major factor in causing obesity. Of the investigators who have studied the level of physical activity of lean and obese subjects some have found no significant difference and others have found a lower level of activity in obese subjects which might represent a difference of perhaps 100 kcal/day in energy expenditure. *If all other factors were equal* this difference of 100 kcal could indeed explain the obesity, but there is no reason to believe that other factors *are* equal. I have been unable to find any publication in which obesity was shown to be caused by inactivity, but this does not mean that it is unimportant. For the reasons explained in Section 3.4, it is technically very difficult to make the appropriate measurements with sufficient accuracy to support any firm conclusion on this matter. For example the study of Garry et al. (1955) on 19 miners and 10 clerks was a huge undertaking conducted with meticulous care. The estimated intake of the clerks exceeded their estimated expenditure on average by 240 kcal (1 MJ)/day, and among the miners the apparent positive balance was 370 kcal (1.5 MJ)/day. If the miners had been obese patients and the clerks lean controls this study might have been hailed as a magnificent demonstration of the reason for obesity in miners, but in fact the miners were not obese, nor were they inactive.

The use of exercise in the treatment of obesity is discussed in Chapter 7, Section 7.5.2.

5.3. Prediction of energy expenditure in individuals

The factors affecting energy expenditure have been reviewed above, and the point has been made repeatedly that there is a large variation between the energy cost of the same task in different individuals, and in the resting metabolic rate between individuals and even in the same individual in different circumstances. The obvious corollary is that it is difficult, with any useful accuracy, to predict the energy expenditure of an individual. However, this is a challenge which is taken up from time to time by investigators who devise formulae, based on such factors as the subject's age, sex, weight, basal metabolism and physical activity, by which his energy expenditure can be computed.

One of the earliest formulae for calculating a "performance index" was that of Jolliffe and Alpert (1951). The use and validation of this index is discussed in 7.2.3. This index, like all similar formulae, is derived by adding together a calculated resting energy expenditure, and a calculated expenditure on physical activity, to obtain total energy expenditure; from this total is subtracted the energy content of the diet to obtain an estimated energy deficit; it is then assumed that this energy deficit is met by loss of tissue which provides 7700 kcal (32.2 MJ)/kg; hence the weight loss on a given reducing diet can be calculated. There are several difficulties with this procedure, some of which are recognised by the originators of the formulae, and some apparently are not.

The first, and most generally recognised, problem is that the weight of the subject affects the calculated energy expenditure, and hence the energy deficit on a given diet. Jolliffe and Alpert overcame this difficulty by recalculating the index for obese patients each time they lost 25 lb (11.3 kg). Recently, however, Antonetti (1973) has proposed a set of equations "easily programmed for a digital computer" whereby this factor is allowed for in the original calculation. The paper of Antonetti will be considered in some detail, since it is based on "an engineering approach to the analysis of the problem of weight change in human beings". This approach involves some formidable mathematics which may well deter the average clinician from too close an inspection of the underlying assumptions. To avoid any similar deterrent effect in this commentary the author's mathematical notation will not be used.

Antonetti's formula (1) states that the change in the total body energy stores is the difference between the amount of energy absorbed from the food, and the amount of energy used for work and lost as heat: at least this is almost what formula (1) says. Had it said exactly this it would have been true, but for some reason the energy derived from food is multiplied by a factor, "an allowance for the specific dynamic action of food", so the change of energy stores is in fact less than the difference between energy going in and energy coming out, which is plainly untrue. Furthermore no indication is given about how this factor to allow for specific dynamic action should be calculated: in worked examples later in the paper it is assumed to be 10%, but no reasons are given for chosing this figure. The argument proceeds with the observation, "It is well known that energy and mass are mutually convertible, and that physiologically, when there is a discrepancy between calorie intake and expenditure, a change in body weight occurs." The observation that a change in body weight is related to energy imbalance is, of course, true, but it has nothing to do with the interconvertibility of mass and energy. When body weight is lost there is no change in the total mass or energy in the universe: carbon and hydrogen in the tissues combine with oxygen from the atmosphere to form carbon dioxide and water in an exothermic reaction. (The effect when mass is converted to energy is outside the limits of physiology since the release of energy is large: this fact is well demonstrated in nuclear explosions.)

In order to derive the energy cost of activity and basal metabolism Antonetti (1973) provides tables from which the appropriate values can be read. In the case of activity the assumption is made that the energy cost of activity is directly related to body weight: that is, a person weighing 100 kg will use twice as much energy for a given level of physical activity as a person who is equally active, but weighs 50 kg. This assumption is totally unfounded. In measurements of the energy cost of stepping up and down a step 25 cm high at the rate of 10 steps/min, Mahadeva et al. (1953) found the energy cost was proportional to $0.66 \times$ weight. Other investigators have found even less effect of body weight on the cost of exercise, and a high level of variability (see 5.1.2). Antonetti (1973) also assumes that the energy cost of resting metabolism is proportional to either surface area or weight to the power of 0.73: the fallacies of this calculation have been discussed in 5.1.

On theoretical grounds, therefore, Antonetti's analysis is open to question. By way of validation he checks his equations against the calculated requirements of the "reference" man and woman postulated by the National Academy of Sciences: agreement is good. This is not surprising, since the requirements of the reference man and woman were derived by similar mathematical processes to those which Antonetti proposes. However, he also shows that his equations fit quite well the mean weight loss of the subjects studied in the Minnesota experiment of experimental semi-starvation (Keys et al., 1950). Again this may be explained by the fact that, in the design of the Minnesota experiment, it was decided to undernourish the volunteers in such a way that their weight fell along a predetermined curve. To do this it was necessary to feed an average of 1570 kcal (6.56 MJ) daily for 24 weeks, in order to achieve a weight loss of about 25% of initial body weight. Assuming a constant intake of 1570 kcal (6.56 MJ), and with subsidiary assumptions about level of physical activity, the Antonetti formula fits the Minnesota weight curve quite well. However this does not show that the Antonetti formula (equation

10) "can be used to calculate weight change as a function of time for a particular caloric intake", as the author's summary suggests, since in the Minnesota experiment the energy intake varied with time for the group as a whole, and individuals varied within the group. For example the mean intake of 1570 kcal over the whole period of 24 weeks was made up of a mean intake of 1658, 1639, 1525, 1434 and 1642 kcal daily for weeks 1, 6, 12, 18 and 24, respectively. Furthermore while the mean intake for the group at week 24 was 1642 kcal, some individuals required about 2000 kcal/day at this stage of the experiment to maintain their weight in parallel with that of the group.

The argument given in favour of the Antonetti formula for estimating weight loss, instead of the "classical" method, is that it is said to be more accurate when the energy deficit is small. An example is given, to illustrate this point, in which a man is fed a diet supplying 2100 kcal (8.8 MJ) when his initial energy requirements are estimated to be 2470 kcal (10.3 MJ) daily. It should be clear from the discussion above that any formula, however computerised, will not estimate energy expenditure with an accuracy better than 15%, since the underlying assumptions are invalid at this level of accuracy. Since the estimate of energy expenditure is liable to be wrong by at least 15%, and the estimate of energy intake also is liable to similar errors (see Chapter 3), it is obvious that an estimated rate of weight loss in an individual subject, based on energy deficits of the order of 15%, is nonsense. If the estimated energy requirement of the subject is 2470 kcal/day, it is likely that the true energy requirement will be somewhere between 2100 and 2800 kcal/day. If the estimated intake on a freely chosen diet is 2100 kcal/day, the true value will probably lie between 1900 and 2300 kcal/day, assuming fairly good dietetic supervision. Thus the energy balance in this hypothetical subject might be anywhere between a deficit of 900 kcal/day and an excess of 200 kcal/day. Therefore, it is impossible to predict accurately even the direction of weight change, and far less possible to calculate the magnitude of the weight change in a given time. The performance index of Jolliffe and Alpert (1951) works fairly well when the difference between estimated intake and expenditure is large, since in this situation errors in the estimation of intake and requirement have relatively less effect on the magnitude of the calculated energy deficit (see 7.2.3).

5.4. Summary: Factors causing differences in energy expenditure between individuals, and changes in individuals

The main message of this chapter is that habitual daily energy expenditure varies considerably between individuals, it is difficult to measure with accuracy (see Chapter 3) and still more difficult to predict (see Section 5.3 above). In order to try to give a general picture of the factors affecting energy output it may be useful to stand back a bit from the uncertainties and technical difficulties of the subject and indulge in some broad generalisation. Concerning differences between individuals I have tried to do this in Fig. 5.8 which shows the probable daily energy expenditure of 6 individuals.

The average sedentary male (for example a clerk) will expend about 2800 kcal (11.7 MJ) daily. This is shown as the top bar in Fig. 5.8 and the hatched area about this mean shows that about 70% of such men will expend on average between 2400 and 3200 kcal, but it should be possible to find such men who would extend the range

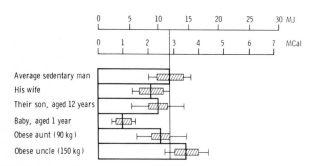

Fig. 5.8. Typical energy expenditure of 6 individuals. An average sedentary man might expend 2800 kcal (11.7 MJ) daily, a group of such men will generally lie in the range indicated by the shaded area, but some will expend as little as 2000 kcal or as much as 3600 kcal/day. Average expenditure with the range similarly indicated is shown for a woman of normal weight, a boy of 12 years, a baby aged 1 year, and an obese woman and man.

from 2000 to 3600 kcal/day. A similar assessment of this man's wife gives an average expenditure of about 2100 kcal (8.8 MJ) with a common range of 1600–2500, and rarely from 1250 to 2800 kcal/day. Their son aged 12 would probably use 2300 kcal on average, but the range in such children is large, so say 2000–2700 commonly and 1200–3400 kcal occasionally. Their baby aged 1 year is assigned an average expenditure of 1000 kcal with a range from 600 to 1500 kcal. An obese aunt, weighing 90 kg, is assigned 2500 kcal with a wide range, and an even more obese uncle weighing 150 kg 3500 kcal, also with a wide range. For reasons explained in Chapter 3.3, it would be very difficult to document these estimates, but I believe both the indicated mean values and the ranges are fairly accurate.

Fig. 5.9 is intended to show the changes in average energy expenditure which might be caused by various events in the life of our average sedentary male. The top bar shows that if he elected to eat his food as a single meal each day, or as 5 meals/day, or if he took on a job with greater administrative responsibilities and worries, this probably would not alter his energy expenditure from its original

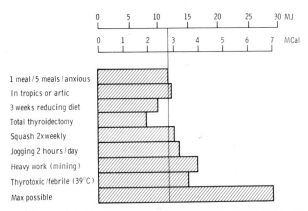

Fig. 5.9. Effect of various conditions on the daily energy expenditure of the average man postulated in Fig. 5.8. Nibbling, gorging and anxiety have no measurable effect on energy expenditure. Underfeeding and thyroidectomy decrease energy expenditure, and climatic extremes and various degrees of physical activity would increase it roughly as indicated. An output of 7000 kcal (29 MJ) in one day would result in exhaustion, and could not be repeated the next day. About 4300 kcal (18 MJ) is a maximum for continuous work.

level of 2800 kcal/day. If he moved to a very hot or very cold climate, but dressed appropriately, he might increase his output by about 5%, mainly due to the effect of heavy clothing in a cold climate making movement more difficult. If he went on a strict reducing diet for 3 weeks his expenditure would probably fall by about 15%, and if he had a total thyroidectomy it would fall about 30%. If he joined the local squash club and played twice a week this might increase output by 10% on average, and 2 h of jogging every evening would cost an extra 400 kcal or so — about a 15% increase. If he lost his clerical job and had to take a strenuous manual job — for example working at the coalface with a pickaxe — his output would rise to about 4000 kcal/day, an increase of 43% on his former occupation. If he developed severe thyrotoxicosis he might have an output of 3600 kcal, an increase of 30%. Finally if he became an Olympic ski racer competing in the 24-h cross-country race, which is probably the greatest of all tests of human fitness and endurance, he might achieve an output of 7000 kcal (29 MJ) in a day, and would then be exhausted, since this is the upper limit of daily energy expenditure. If, less happily, he fell overboard in cold seas he might by shivering thermogenesis achieve a similar heat output for a day, but one hopes that he would then be rescued, since he could not repeat the performance for another day.

CHAPTER 6

Energy stores: their composition, measurement and control

A normal rat achieves quite an accurate matching between energy intake and energy expenditure each day, while normal man does not. This is illustrated in Fig. 6.1, taken from the data of Edholm et al. (1955). The normal young men they studied often expended 1000 kcal (4.2 MJ) more or less than they ate during the same day, so the imbalance had to be met by adding to, or subtracting from, the energy stores of the body.

6.1. Body weight and its components

Body weight is easy to measure to one hundredth of one per cent with a simple beam balance, but the weight of the body bears no simple relationship to the size of the energy stores, nor is a change in energy stores necessarily reflected in a change in weight. Under carefully controlled conditions in a subject who is close to energy balance it is possible to obtain the relationship shown in Fig. 2.2. In this case small imbalances between intake and output are being met from the glycogen stores of the body. However, when large imbalances occur the excess or deficit is balanced by changes in the store of adipose tissue, which has a much higher energy density. Therefore it is necessary to know the nature of the energy store which is being changed before weight change can be interpreted in terms of energy balance.

6.1.1. Body composition determined by direct analysis

Our understanding of the composition of the human body is based on chemical analyses of 6 cadavers which were performed between

114

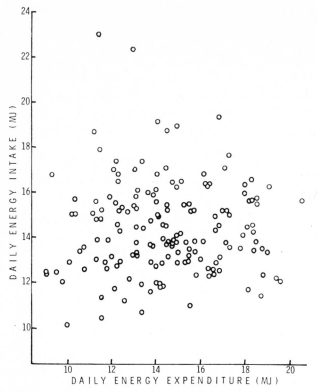

Fig. 6.1. Daily energy intake of 12 cadets over a period of 14 days, plotted against the daily energy expenditure of the same individual on the same day (from Edholm et al., 1955).

1945 and 1956. Mitchell et al. (1945) analysed a 35-year-old white male who died suddenly of a heart attack. Widdowson et al. (1951) analysed two adults and a child: the adults were a man of 25 who died of uraemia and a woman of 42 who drowned herself. Forbes et al. (1953) analysed a man of 46 who died of a fractured skull, and Forbes et al. (1956) reported two more analyses: one of a Negro male with bacterial endocarditis who died aged 48, and the other a man of 60 who was found dead, presumably of a heart attack. Further data on the electrolyte composition of the last two bodies was published by Forbes and Lewis (1956). The composition of individual organs has been extensively investigated by Dickerson and Widdowson (1960) and Widdowson and Dickerson (1960).

It is obviously not practicable to measure the energy stores of a patient by direct chemical analysis, so various indirect methods have been developed, which are discussed later in this chapter. These all to a greater or lesser degree rest on the assumption that the body consists of two components: fat, and lean tissue of a fairly constant composition. The limitations of this approach are indicated in Table 6.1, which shows the water, protein and potassium concentration of the fat-free bodies which were analysed by the investigators mentioned above. It can be seen that each kilogramme of fat-free tissue contains about 725 g water, 205 g protein, and 69 mmoles potassium, but that there is considerable variation between the individual bodies. In the lower part of Table 6.1 the composition of various organs is shown, and it is obvious that fat-free skin, for example, has a very different water and potassium content from, say, brain or muscle. It

TABLE 6.1

THE CONTRIBUTION OF WATER AND PROTEIN TO THE FAT-FREE WEIGHT OF 6 ADULT BODIES, AND IN SOME ORGANS (for sources of these data see text)

	Age (years)	Water (g/kg)	Protein (g/kg)	Remainder (g/kg)	Potassium (mmoles/kg)	K : N ratio (mmoles/g)
Fat-free whole bodies						
	25	728	195	77	71.5	2.29
	35	775	165	60	—	—
	42	733	192	75	73.0	2.38
	46	674	234	92	66.5	1.78
	48	730	206	64	—	—
	60	704	238	58	66.6	1.75
Mean		725	205	71	69.0	2.05
Selected organs						
Skin		694	300	6	23.7	0.45
Heart		827	143	30	66.5	2.90
Liver		711	176	113	75.0	2.66
Kidneys		810	153	37	57.0	2.33
Brain		774	107	119	84.6	4.96
Muscle		792	192	16	92.2	2.99

116

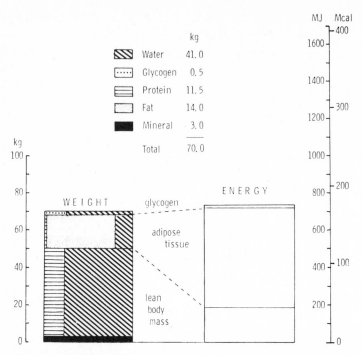

Fig. 6.2. The body composition of a normal adult male who weighs 70 kg. The diagram on the left indicates the approximate composition of lean body mass and adipose tissue in terms of the weight of water, protein, fat and mineral, while the diagram on the right shows the equivalent energy value of these components. The glycogen—water pool is assumed to be 2 kg.

is possible to illustrate the energy stores associated with moderately severe obesity by means of the simplified models shown in Figs. 6.2 and 6.3. Fig. 6.2 shows the relationship of body composition to energy stores in a normal 70-kg man. Water is the main component of body weight, but contributes nothing to the energy store. Adipose tissue in this model consists of 14 kg fat, 3.5 kg water and 0.5 kg protein, making 18 kg out of the total weight of 70 kg, but by far the greatest proportion of the energy stores is derived from this adipose tissue. The glycogen—water pool is assumed to be 2 kg, of which 0.5 kg is glycogen and 1.5 kg water, since this is roughly the proportions in which these two are stored (Olsson and Saltin, 1970).

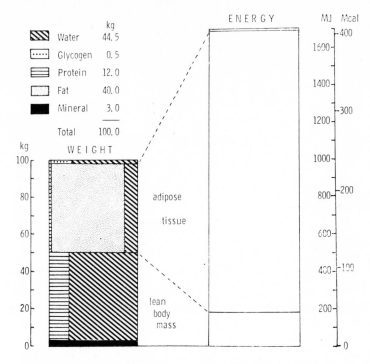

Fig. 6.3. The body composition of an obese adult male who weighs 100 kg. The lean body mass and glycogen pool have been assumed to be similar to that of the subject shown in Fig. 6.2. The extra weight is due to an extra 30 kg of adipose tissue, which has increased the energy stores by approximately 1000 MJ.

If the hypothetical subject shown in Fig. 6.2 became obese by acquiring an extra 30 kg of adipose tissue his weight and energy stores would resemble the situation shown in Fig. 6.3. For simplicity it is assumed that the size and composition of the lean tissue would be unchanged, but in practice this is not so, which causes problems discussed further in Section 6.2.2. The important point illustrated in Fig. 6.3 is that an increase in weight from 70 kg to 100 kg is associated with an increase in energy stores from 174 Mcal (736 MJ) to 410 Mcal (1715 MJ). If this obese person is able to maintain a negative energy balance of 500 kcal (2.1 MJ) daily it would take him 16 months to reduce his energy stores to their former state.

6.1.2. Fluctuations in body weight

The point has already been made in Section 4.4 that body weight in normal individuals is not very constant (as is often claimed) but tends to show long-term oscillations of about 10 kg from year to year. However, of much greater importance to the obese patient trying to lose weight are the fickle fluctuations of a few hundred grammes from day to day. Anyone who deals with obese patients knows the despair caused by a slight increase in weight not explicable by any known departure from the prescribed diet. Often these minor fluctuations are so distressing that the doctor is forced to take refuge in explanations which he does not believe himself: there is vague mention of "glandular disturbance" or "fluid retention" (see Section 2.2.2).

Of course there are fluctuations in body weight even in patients who are fed a precisely controlled diet in a metabolic ward, but they are small. Fig. 6.4 shows the daily weights of a patient in our ward who was fed 1000 kcal (4.2 MJ) during the first and third week of her admission, and 500 kcal (2.1 MJ) during the second week. There

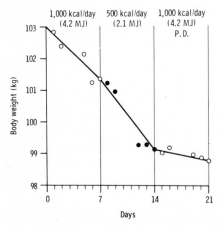

Fig. 6.4. Daily weight of an obese patient fed a constant diet in a metabolic ward. Note the small daily variation about the trend line and the slower rate of weight loss in the week on 1000 kcal after one on 500 kcal, compared with that in the first week.

is some scatter of the points about the line showing the general trend in weight, but never more than 0.5 kg deviation.

In people who are taking a diet varying in salt and carbohydrate content, and who have varying patterns of exercise, daily weight is less stable and less obviously related to the energy content of the diet. Adam et al. (1961) made over 1700 measurements of weight in 64 soldiers and found a change of more than 0.5 kg in a day on 30% of readings, and 1.0 kg in 5% of readings, and similar results were obtained in an even larger series of measurements by Edholm et al. (1974). Weight of faeces passed does not explain these fluctuations. Khosla and Billewicz (1964) obtained similar results on 19 subjects weighed daily for 30–40 days.

The effect of menstruation on weight was investigated by Robinson and Watson (1965) who weighed 28 female students who had an average premenstrual weight gain of 300 g and reached a minimum weight on the eighth day of the menstrual cycle. Taggart (1962) found no significant relationship of weight to her menstrual cycle over an observation period of 80 days.

6.1.3. Energy equivalence of weight loss

Weight loss may be of zero energy value (as when water is lost under the influence of a diuretic), or at maximum 9000 kcal (3.8 MJ)/ kg if pure fat was entirely responsible for the weight loss. In practice the energy value of weight loss in obese patients on a reducing diet tends to increase as weight loss proceeds. In Fig. 2.2 the energy value of weight change is about 1000 kcal (4.2 MJ)/kg, since this is the energy value of 250 g glycogen with 750 g water bound to it. If the subject continues in negative energy balance the glycogen stores become depleted, so the energy deficit must be met to a greater extent either by fat or by lean tissue. Passmore et al. (1958) made a detailed study of the composition of weight loss in 7 patients who were fed a diet supplying only about 400 kcal daily for 6 weeks. This study has been reviewed in detail (Garrow, 1974b), and it shows very well the initial loss of glycogen and water, followed by a period during which fat was the main fuel used to supply the energy deficit, so over the whole 6-week period the calculated average energy value of the tissue loss was calculated to be between 7000 and 8000 kcal/kg for the 7 subjects.

Dole et al. (1955) alternately overfed or underfed 5 obese patients by 485 kcal/day for 4 days. The experiment continued for 32 days and included 4 overfeeding and 4 underfeeding periods. Since the imbalance was nearly 2000 kcal it was not to be expected that this could be met entirely from the glycogen pool, and indeed the calculated energy equivalence of the weight gained or lost in this study was about 2000 kcal/kg, which suggests that it was partly glycogen and partly fat which was being burned and replaced.

The results of an investigation to see if exercise altered the energy equivalence of weight loss are shown in Fig. 6.5. Fourteen obese women were given a diet supplying 800 kcal (3.4 MJ) daily for 3 weeks, and their average daily weight loss was plotted against their energy deficit. Energy deficit was calculated by subtracting energy

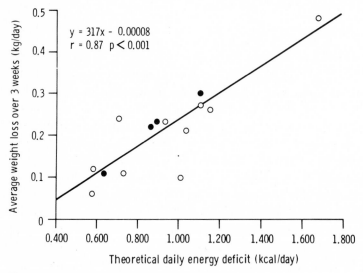

Fig. 6.5. Average daily weight loss in 14 obese women on a diet supplying 800 kcal (3.4 MJ) daily for 3 weeks. The theoretical daily energy deficit was calculated by subtracting intake from measured energy expenditure. The 4 patients shown by filled circles also undertook daily exercise, but this did not affect their rate of weight loss.

intake from energy expenditure measured by indirect calorimetry. Four of the women also undertook exercise daily on a treadmill or bicycle ergometer in order to expend an extra 300 kcal (1.2 MJ) daily: these are shown on Fig. 6.5 as filled circles, while the patients not taking extra exercise are shown as open circles. There is (as expected) a good correlation between weight loss and energy deficit, but this relationship was no different in the exercising women.

It is possible from the data in Fig. 6.5 to calculate the energy equivalent of weight loss for each patient, and it can be seen that it ranges from about 3000 to 6000 kcal/kg, which is the result to be expected in the light of the discussion above. The patient shown in Fig. 6.4 had an energy expenditure of about 2000 kcal (8.4 MJ) daily, so overall her weight loss of 4.2 kg represents an energy deficit of about 25,000 kcal in the 3 weeks, or 6000 kcal/kg, but during the first week it was much less, and in the last week much more, than this average figure. Thus it is necessary to be careful in interpreting the energy value of weight loss over short periods, especially when the diet is being changed.

6.2. Adipose tissue

It is quite a simple matter to obtain a sample of subcutaneous adipose tissue from a patient, either by needle biopsy (Hirsch and Goldrick, 1964) or by open surgical biopsy. Many investigators have analysed such samples, with the results which are summarised in Table 6.2. In lean subjects subcutaneous adipose tissue is about 18% water, 3% protein and 79% fat, but in obese subjects the fat cells are more tightly packed with fat, so the proportions are about 14% water, 2% protein and 84% fat. These figures are obviously approximate, since the analytical results will be influenced by the amount of stromal tissue which is included in the sample, and there is no easy way of differentiating adipose tissue from its supporting connective tissue. The problems of measuring the size and number of fat cells, and interpreting the results of these measurements, are considered further in Section 6.2.3.

TABLE 6.2

THE CHEMICAL COMPOSITION OF SUBCUTANEOUS ADIPOSE TISSUE

PM = post-mortem examination.

Author	Biopsy (n) or PM	Water %		Fat %		Protein %		Weight
		Mean	Range or ±S.D.	Mean	Range or ±S.D.	Mean	Range or ±S.D.	
Entenman et al. (1958)	Biopsy "B" "E"	32.4 17.7		62.3 78.9		—		86.6 kg 80.7 kg
Pawan and Clode (1960)	Biopsy (6) PM (14)	28.6 26.1	(18.2–50.6) (9.6–53.0)	68.4 72.1	(61.4–82.4) (42.8–85.9)	2.1 —	(1.8–2.8)	lean lean
Thomas (1962)	Biopsy (41)	14.2	(6.6–36.1)	82.3	(61.0–92.4)	2.9	(1.1–6.5)	<110%
Morse and Soeldner (1963)	Biopsy (17)	15.4	±4.8	—		—		lean
Baker (1969)	PM (4) (10)	19.7 18.8		— —		1.9 2.1		(age 19–25 years) (age 38–71 years)
Weighted mean for 94 lean subjects		18.1		78.3		2.6		
Entenman et al. (1958)	Biopsy "B" "E"	18.0 12.5		79.2 85.7		— —		101.5 kg 89.1 kg
Pawan and Clode (1960)	Biopsy (7) PM (14)	18.8 14.6	(12.7–30.1) (6.7–28.9)	78.7 78.8	(67.0–85.1) (66.6–91.0)	2.0 —	(1.8–2.7)	obese obese
Thomas (1962)	Biopsy (20)	10.0	(4.4–14.1)	87.6	(78.2–94.1)	2.4	(1.0–4.4)	>110%
Morse and Soeldner (1963)	Biopsy (12)	15.1	±5.2	—		—		obese
Weighted mean for 55 obese subjects		13.6		83.2		2.3		

6.2.1. Measurement of total body fat by fat-soluble gases or skinfolds

All anaesthetic gases are very soluble in fat: this general rule probably means that their anaesthetic action requires interaction with some functional lipid in the nervous system. However, it is possible to use this property to make a direct estimate of the total fat content of a living subject. This approach has been used by Hytten et al. (1966) using krypton as the marker gas, and Lesser et al. (1971) have used both radioactive krypton and cyclopropane. Although the method is theoretically excellent it is difficult to use in practice (Halliday, 1971), because the subject has to breathe in a leak-free closed circuit apparatus until an equilibrium is set up between the partial pressure of the marker gas in the air mixture and in all body fat. This takes a long time, because these gases are very soluble in fat, but relatively inefficiently transported in the bloodstream from the lungs to the adipose depots. If all fat depots were equally and uniformly perfused with blood it might be possible to predict the eventual equilibrium situation on the basis of the early rate of uptake. However, hopes of this sort are dashed by the demonstration that the blood flow in human subcutaneous adipose tissue shows a coefficient of variation of 62% between subjects, 35% between successive measurements on the same subject, and 10% between simultaneous measurements at symmetrical points on a single subject (Bulow et al., 1976). With so fickle a system it would obviously be unwise to attempt to predict the eventual equilibrium concentration from measurements during, for example, the first 30 min of the uptake curve. Furthermore there is no reason to believe that the perfusion of adipose tissue in obese patients obeys the same laws as that in lean people, or that it would remain unchanged if the obese patient lost a substantial amount of adipose tissue.

We must therefore regretfully conclude that measurement of total body fat by fat-soluble gases is unlikely to be clinically useful so long as it depends on the patient breathing the marker gas until a steady state is reached.

A much more convenient method for measuring fatness is with skinfold calipers. Many authors have pointed out that most of the fat stored in the body lies under the skin (Edwards, 1950) and that the thickness of a fold of skin picked up at strategic sites indicates the amount of subcutaneous fat (Montoye et al., 1965; Seltzer and Mayer, 1965). Various sites for measurement have been suggested: Hermansen and Von Döbeln (1971) used 11 sites, Strakova and Markova (1971) 15 sites, and Seltzer and Mayer (1965) relied only on a single skinfold over the triceps. However, probably the best established system is that using 4 sites: biceps, triceps, subscapular and suprailiac. These were proposed by Durnin and Rahaman (1967) and developed by Durnin et al. (1971), Durnin and Womersley (1974) and Womersley and Durnin (1977) to include standards based on 245 men and 324 women covering the age range from 17 to 72 years. Fat-free mass (calculated from skinfolds) agrees well with total body nitrogen (measured by neutron activation analysis). Hill et al. (1978) found a coefficient of variation of 8.5% between the two measurements.

However, measurement of skinfolds requires skill and training. Ruiz et al. (1971) showed that it was important that the triceps skinfold was measured at exactly the correct site, otherwise false results were obtained. In very fat people it is impossible to obtain a true fold of skin and subcutaneous fat, and if you do so it will not fit between the jaws of the standard caliper. Attempts have been made to measure the thickness of the subcutaneous fat layer by X-rays (Garn, 1961; Tanner, 1965) or by ultrasound (Booth et al., 1966; Hawes et al., 1972; Haymes et al., 1976) but these techniques are less convenient than skinfold caliper measurements with little compensating advantage. A theoretical limitation to the skinfold measurement is that it assumes a constant relationship between subcutaneous and deep fat stores, which is not confirmed by measurement at post-mortem examinations (Alexander, 1964), but the tables of Durnin and Womersley (1974) give different standards for percentage body fat according to age and sex, which to some extent compensates for age- and sex-related changes in the distribution of fat in the body. Jones et al. (1976) found differences between the proportion of fat which was subcutaneous in Europeans, Gurkhas, Rajputs and South Indians, so there are also probably ethnic differences which should be considered when converting from skinfold thickness measurements to estimates of body fat. Despite these reservations skinfolds are certainly the most convenient method for estimating fat in people of reasonably normal build, provided that the measurements are made by a trained observer and an error of about 3% of body weight (i.e. 2 kg of fat in an average subject) is acceptable. This is probably the error in skilled hands (Durnin and Womersley, 1977). In unskilled hands, and with fatter subjects, the error will be much greater, but this does not prevent some authors from applying the method in circumstances which are quite inappropriate. The paper by Grimes and Franzini (1977), for example, comes from a department of psychology, so one cannot be sure that it is not an elaborate hoax. They suggest that skinfolds should be used to "measure change in behavioural weight control studies", and explain, with diagrams, how to take measurements at the sites used by Durnin and Rahaman (1967). They note the "lack of normative data for extremely or morbidly obese patients" but solve this difficulty with a stroke of the pen: since the standards of Durnin and Rahaman stop at a total skinfold reading of 95 mm they simply extend the line to 150 mm! If this paper is intended as a humorous parody of the way skinfolds are misused the authors have done brilliantly. If (as I fear) it is a serious contribution they should be strongly advised to offer their calipers in part exchange for some bathroom scales, which would provide a much better "measure of change in behavioural weight control studies".

6.2.2. Measurement of lean body mass by water or potassium

Total body fat is difficult to measure accurately for the reasons explained above. However, if it were possible to measure the mass of lean tissue in a living subject, his fat mass could easily be calculated by subtracting lean mass from total body weight. McCance and Widdowson (1951) described "a method of breaking down the body weights of living persons into terms of extracellular fluid, cell mass and fat, . . .", Behnke et al. (1942) proposed the ratio of body weight to volume as an index of obesity, while as early as 1938 Talbot (1938) was measuring obesity in children by their daily creatinine excretion. With advances in techniques for detecting radiation Burch and Spiers (1953) were able to detect the radiation coming from the natural radioactive isotope of potassium ^{40}K, and thus estimate the potassium content of living subjects, while more recently still neutron activation (Cohn et al., 1974, 1976) has made it possible to measure induced radioactivity in quite a large range of elements in the human body. All these approaches depend on some assumed relationship between the thing measured (water, density, creatinine excretion or potassium) and the mass of lean tissue in the body.

The most used methods, which will be discussed here, involve measurement of total body water or total body potassium, and some factor to convert this to mass of lean tissue. Only the modern techniques in current use will be reviewed here, but readers who are interested in the development of the techniques will find historical reviews in the publications cited above or in Garrow (1974b).

Pace and Rathbun (1945) measured the water content of the fat-free bodies of 50 eviscerated guinea pigs and found that it was 72.4% with a standard deviation of 2.11%. They did not claim in that paper that the water content of the fat-free bodies of guinea pigs was independent of the fatness of the animal, although this conclusion has been ascribed to them. In fact careful review of their results shows that the 5 thinnest animals had an average water content of 68.7% of fat-free weight, while the fattest 5 animals average 72.7%. However, the average value found by Pace and Rathbun in guinea pigs and other species agrees well with the average value of 72.5% in fat-free human bodies (see Table 6.1), so it is reasonable to expect that if total body water can be measured in man this will give a reliable estimate of fat-free mass, and by subtraction of this from body weight total body fat can be calculated.

Luckily, it is quite easy to measure total body water in man. A dose of water labelled with either deuterium oxide or tritium oxide is given and it equilibrates with water in all the body fluids in about 4 h. If a sample of any body fluid (but most conveniently blood) is taken, after this equilibrium condition has been achieved, the dilution of the administered dose can be calculated and hence the volume in which the dose was distributed. This is almost equal to total body water: about 2% of labelled hydrogen ions exchange with labile organic hydrogen atoms to give a slightly high apparent volume of distribution, but this source of error is not in practice very important (Culebras et al., 1977).

Very accurate measurement of total body water can be achieved using the technique of Halliday and Miller (1977), but scrupulous attention to procedural detail is needed if errors are not to creep in to the estimation. There are 5 stages at which poor technique may give a false answer. First it is necessary to measure the administered dose with an accuracy of about 0.1%. This is not difficult if the deuterated water is injected and the injection syringe is weighed before and after giving the dose, or alternatively if the labelled water is taken by mouth diluted in about 70 g tap water (Halliday and Miller, 1977) it must be drunk through a straw, and the container and straw are weighed before and after giving the dose. Next it is necessary to measure the amount of labelled water lost during the equilibration period, since the effective dose at equilibrium is that remaining in the body at the time when the equilibrium sample is taken. The third point is that two samples of body fluid (usually blood) are required to measure the increase in concentration of deuterium resulting from the administered dose. The variation in deuterium concentration in the blood of different people, or even between water from urine, plasma, serum, saliva and expired air in the same person (Halliday and Miller, 1977), is such that a sample of the same fluid must be taken before, as well as after, the dose is given. The fourth source of error is that complete equilibration of the labelled water with body water may not be achieved, either because too short a time was allowed for equilibration, or alternatively because the patient (unknown to the investigator) drank some unlabelled water shortly before the "equilibrated" blood sample was taken, and thus upset the uniform distribution of the label. Finally great care is needed in the analysis of the sample, especially to ensure that while it is being converted from water to a mixture of hydrogen and deuterium gas for mass spectrometry the ratio of the hydrogen isotopes is not altered. These aspects, and the technical problems of mass spectrometry of hydrogen gas, are discussed by Halliday and Miller (1977).

It is difficult to achieve all these steps with an accuracy of better than 1% using tritiated water, since the statistics of counting a sample of body fluid after an ethically acceptable radiation dose of tritium place a severe limit on the accuracy of the method. Nielsen et al. (1971) describe a method with a rather large dose of deuterium (approximately 100 g per subject) and using gas chromatography to measure the concentration of isotope in serum. They claim that this gives an answer for total body water in man accurate to 0.5 litre, but it is difficult to accept this estimate since measurements of standard solutions by gas chromatography in their hands were associated with errors of 3%. By contrast, isotope mass spectrometry requires a dose of only 1–2 g deuterium oxide, it has a sensitivity of 2 parts in 10^7, requires a sample of 5 μl for measurement and typically gives replicate measurements on standard samples in this range which agree within 0.05%.

Given facilities for high precision isotope mass spectrometry it is possible to measure total body water to better than 0.5 litre, but the problem of converting this measurement to an estimate of fat-free mass remains. Among the 50 eviscerated guinea pigs analysed by Pace and Rathbun (1945) the fat-free body had a water content of 72.4% with a standard deviation of 2.11%, and the results summarised in Table 6.1 suggest that an equal variability in hydration occurs in fat-free human bodies. Indeed Womersley et al. (1976) and Wang and Pierson (1976) provide direct evidence that the hydration of the fat-free body in man is inconstant.

The measurement of total body potassium offers an alternative method for estimating the amount of lean tissue in living subjects, but with this method also points of technique are important. A gamma spectrometer which will make an accurate measurement of the radiation from the natural isotope ^{40}K in a human body is an expensive piece of equipment: it needs expert maintenance and a massive shield to protect it as far as possible from interference from cosmic radiation and other sources of background radioactivity. Some publications which compare potassium measurements unfavourably with other methods of estimating body fat are hardly fair to the technique, since the equipment used for potassium measurement is so inferior. For example Chien et al. (1975) conclude that skinfolds and density measurements are better than potassium counting, which is not surprising since they were using a single NaI crystal 8 in. in diameter to measure potassium. Such a counter would be perfectly satisfactory for identifying very low levels of radioactive contaminants in a human subject, but it can hardly give an estimate of total body potassium in a 40-min counting period with an error less than 8%. The design and calibration of gamma spectrometers are outside the scope of this book, but to interpret total body potassium results it is necessary to know something about the measuring apparatus. Installations with an array of many detectors surrounding the subject are more likely to give a reliable answer than those which rely on a constant proportion of the radiation from the subject hitting a single detector. Even with the most expensive and sophisticated installations it is very difficult to reduce measurement error below 3%, and different counters give different answers despite all efforts to calibrate them. For example Ellis et al. (1974) are very experienced workers in this field, but report that the Brookhaven counter gave answers which were on average 4.4% lower than those obtained for the same subjects on the installation at St. Luke's Medical Centre.

The accuracy with which a gamma spectrometer measures total body potassium can be determined by counting the ^{40}K radiation, and then checking the result by chemical analysis of the body. This has been done in monkeys by Kodama et al. (1974) and in children by Garrow (1965b), but so far as I know never in adult humans.

Having obtained an estimate of potassium, problems of interpretation arise similar to those discussed above with water estimations. An interesting demonstration that the lean tissue of obese patients cannot maintain a constant proportion of water and potassium is shown in Fig. 6.6. If each kilogramme of fat-free tissue contained 725 g of water and 69 mmoles of potassium (to take the average figures from Table 6.1) then every patient, however obese, must have a water/potassium ratio of 10.51. In women the potassium concentration is probably nearer 60 mmoles/kg fat-free tissue, so the ratio might be about 12 g water/mmole of potassium. Among patients of fairly normal weight measured at the Clinical Research Centre in England a ratio of about 12 is found, but as patients become more obese the ratio becomes higher and more variable. The open circles on Fig. 6.6 relate to very obese patients studied by Bray et al. (1970), and it is obvious that the assumption of a constant proportion of water and potassium in the fat-free tissue of these patients cannot possibly be valid.

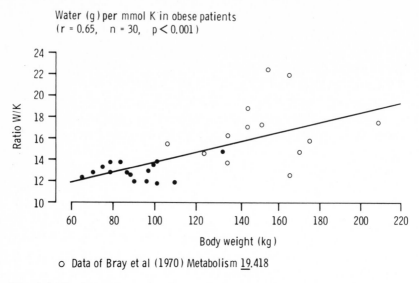

Fig. 6.6. The increasing ratio of water to potassium in very obese patients.

So far the best solution to this problem is that used by Berg and Isaksson (1970) who measure both water and potassium in their patients and calculate body composition using a set of assumptions which, although rather arbitrary, seem to lead to a fairly reliable conclusion. The assumptions are that fat-free extracellular solids account for 12% of body weight, that the body cell mass contains 120 mmoles potassium/kg, and contains 78% of water. The water not accounted for by this intracellular water is extracellular water. Thus the components of body weight by this model are fat-free extracellular solids, body cell mass, extracellular water and fat, and since from measurements of water and potassium the first three of these components can be calculated the fourth, namely fat, can be obtained by subtracting the others from total body weight.

Since the apparatus for measuring total body potassium is expensive to buy and difficult to maintain many attempts have been made to "predict" the answer from simpler measurements, but these shortcuts are not very satisfactory. Certainly total body potassium concentration is not related to erythrocyte potassium concentration (Boddy et al., 1976): it would be surprising if it were so. Forbes

(1974) reviewed the literature on measurements of lean body mass by potassium counting and concluded that in adult men and women it was quite well correlated with height cubed. Ward et al. (1975) measured height, weight, circumference at 5 sites, skinfolds at 2 sites, and diameters at 9 sites on 223 male and 36 female military personnel and concluded that the measurements best correlated with weight of fat in men were waist circumference, weight and buttock circumference, while in women the best correlations were with triceps skinfold and scapular skinfold. In all cases the correlation coefficients between these measurements and estimates of fat by density, potassium or water measurements were around 0.7–0.8. Pollock et al. (1975) measured 8 skinfolds, 13 girths, 7 diameters, age, weight, height and bra cup size in 83 women in an attempt "to increase the predictability of body density" (they say). Correlation equations showed that in younger women the "best fit" to density was given by skinfold at thigh and suprailiac sites, knee diameter and wrist girth ($r = 0.83$). Turner and Cohn (1975) measured the weight, height and age of 31 men, and found that the equation: TBK = 30.83 ht (cm) + 18.05 wt (kg) — 11 (age (years) — 20) — 3034 gave a correlation coefficient of 0.92.

Burkinshaw et al. (1971) propose an equation for men to predict potassium: —42.83 + 1.45 wt + 7.78 thigh muscle width — 5.91 fat width, where the widths of muscle and fat are measured from a radiograph of the thigh. For women the equation is: 4.44 + 0.97 wt + 4.38 muscle — 3.27 fat. Ellis et al. (1974) offer an equation to predict total body potassium which is "custom-fit, based on the individual's physical characteristics of age, sex, weight and height." The formula involves multiplying the square root of the weight (kg) by the square of the height (m) and this by a constant for men of 5.52–0.014 times age in years, and for women the constant is 4.58 — 0.010 times age in years. The standard deviation of the potassium as measured and as predicted by this formula is about 10%. Shizgal (1976) assumes that the ratio of the sum of total body sodium and potassium to the total body water must be constant for all tissues and thus derives total body potassium from measurements of total body water and exchangeable sodium. Spainier and Shizgal (1977) use this method to calculate caloric requirements of critically ill patients, and the answer may well be correct, but the theoretical basis is indeed insecure. It is not too difficult to show that in critically ill patients the ratio of sodium and potassium to water is not constant for all tissues (Garrow, 1965a; Halliday, 1967).

This is not an exhaustive review of equations to "predict" body potassium or density from simpler measurements: other formulae are offered by Steinkamp et al. (1965), Zuti and Golding (1973) and many others. The process of generating "predictive" formulae which are really retrospective will probably go on for ever. For the reasons given in Section 2.6.2 anyone can produce a better predictive formula than everyone else when used retrospectively on their own data. This section will have served some useful function if editors of journals henceforth refuse to publish descriptions of "predictive" formulae unless they are actually shown to work *predictively*.

6.2.3. Measurement of fat cell size and number

The clinical significance of the cellularity of adipose tissue is discussed in Section 7.7.1. However, much of the confusion in the literature has arisen from the technical problems of measuring the size and number of fat cells. This will be briefly considered here.

There are 3 methods commonly used to measure the size of fat cells in a sample of adipose tissue. One is to fix the cells with osmic acid (Hirsch and Gallian, 1968) and count the particles with an electronic counter, another is to free the cells by incubation with collagenase and photograph the resulting suspension of spherical cells (Bray, 1970a), and the third is to examine a fixed section of adipose tissue microscopically (Bjurulf, 1959). A discussion of the relative merits of these methods is given by Sjöström (1976). All the methods depend on the presence of fat in the cells, and in the case of the osmium tetroxide method there has to be quite a lot of fat in the cell for it to be counted. Undoubtedly there are fat cells with very little fat, which can only be seen in fixed sections (Kirtland et al., 1975), and systems using fixed sections are now generally preferred (Ashwell et al., 1975c, 1976). It is still an open question if there are "preadipocytes" which have not stored enough fat to be recognised by any of the methods mentioned above, but that question is out of the scope of the present review.

If we consider only fat cells which actually contain fat, the average size of these cells in a biopsy sample can be determined by the method of Ashwell et al. (1976). Fat cell size varies from site to site in the same person, so to obtain a representative sample it is necessary to take biopsies from several sites (Ashwell et al., 1978). To calculate fat cell number it is necessary to divide total body fat by the average fat per fat cell, and it should be evident from the discussion above that one of the most difficult parts of this calculation is to obtain a reliable estimate of total body fat, especially in a person in whom the fat mass is changing.

Several investigators have reported that fat cell number does not change in an obese patient who loses fat: the cells decrease in size but not in number (Björntorp et al., 1975). On average this seems to be true, but the statement is of the "constancy fallacy" type (see

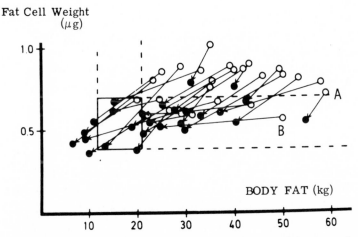

Fig. 6.7. Total body fat and average fat cell size in 26 women before (○) and after (●) weight loss which averaged 15 kg (data of Björntorp et al., 1975). Note that in patient A the decrease in cell size is *greater* than the change in body fat (indicating an increase in fat cell number) and in patient B the reverse is true (indicating a decrease in fat cell number) but that the *average* fat cell number in this group of women is not significantly altered after weight loss.

2.6.1). The data in Fig. 6.7 are taken from the publication by Björn-torp et al. (1975) and shows that 26 women originally had increased body fat and big fat cells (open circles) and when they lost weight the size of their fat cells tended to move into the normal range indicated by the broken lines. However, if it were true that fat cell number is constant during fat loss the loss of fat in each patient should be proportional to the loss of fat in her fat cells: in other words the arrows connecting the open circles (which show the situation at the start of treatment) to the filled circles (which show the situation after weight reduction) should all point towards the origin of the x and y axes of the graph. In fact they do not. Two extreme patients are indicated on the figure: patient A started with about 59 kg of fat, and an average fat cell weight of 0.7 μg, and reduced to about 54 kg of fat, with an average fat cell weight of 0.53 μg. If we now calculate the fat cell number implied by these results it gives an estimate of 8.43×10^{10} fat cells at the time of the first biopsy, and 10.19×10^{10} fat cells after weight loss! At the other extreme patient B apparently had about 50 kg of fat, with a fat cell weight of 0.55 μg before treatment, and 24 kg of fat and a fat cell weight of 0.51 μg after treatment: this implies a change from 9.09×10^{10} to 4.71×10^{10} fat cells. Thus there may be no general change in fat cell number in the group as a whole, but there is certainly a change in the estimated number of fat cells in members of the group.

6.3. Body composition measurements to check estimates of energy balance

It should be evident to the reader who has reached this point that there is no simple relationship between weight change and change in the energy stores of the body. In the treatment of obesity the objective is to reduce the excessive energy stores (mainly fat), but for the reasons given in Section 6.2, it is difficult to measure body fat accurately. If it is measured inaccurately quite incorrect conclusions may be reached about the effectiveness of various types of treatment for obesity. Grande (1968) published a critical review of 3 papers in which investigators had deceived themselves (and presumably the editorial referees in the journals which published their results) by use of inappropriate measures of body composition. It is impertinent to try to precis Grande's masterly analysis: the essential points will be mentioned here. Benoit et al. (1965) concluded that fasting subjects lost only 350 g of fat/day, while if they were given a ketogenic diet providing 1000 kcal (4.2 MJ) daily they lost 640 g fat/day. They arrived at this highly improbable conclusion as a result of a misplaced faith in total body potassium measurements. The study of Bolinger et al. (1966) provides good data on the effects of starvation or 40 g protein on nitrogen balance, but the use of sodium balance to calculate fluid spaces and hence changes in fat leads to improbable estimates of energy expenditure. Ball et al. (1967) put too much faith in estimations of total body water by tritium dilution and also arrive at estimates of energy balance which are highly improbable. Other examples are discussed in some detail by Garrow (1974b) and the problem has recently been reviewed by Yang et al. (1977).

6.3.1. Energy balance and nitrogen balance

It is remarkable that the two most convincing studies of body composition changes in obese patients on a reducing diet are those of Passmore et al. (1958) in Edinburgh, and Yang and Van Itallie (1976) in New York. These two studies are separated by 18 years, 3000 miles and vast changes in the technology associated with the measurement of body composition, but both relied on the same two measurements: nitrogen balance and energy balance. These methods are not widely used, since they are unpopular both with the investigators and the subjects. To perform nitrogen balance accurately it is necessary to have absolute control over the food intake of the subjects, and it is preferable that this food is homogeneous for ease of analysis (see 3.1.1). All excreta must be collected and analysed by the Kjeldahl technique, which is a rather sordid chore for both subjects and investigators. Measurements of energy expenditure and intake involve similar restrictions on movement and invasion of privacy of the subjects. Patients will tolerate conditions normally associated with prisons rather than hospitals for a few weeks if the reasons are carefully explained (Garrow et al., 1978): indeed the procedure most likely to infuriate obese patients is to admit them to a metabolic ward where the patients are allowed a reasonable degree of freedom, and then when they fail to lose weight they are accused of "cheating" on the diet!

There is obviously a need for some method for checking body composition measurement which does not require prolonged imprisonment of the subjects, but the errors associated with the available procedures are such that they are only reliable if large weight changes are produced, and perhaps not even then (Pierson et al., 1976). If large weight changes are to be monitored by accurate measurements of energy balance this still requires prolonged imprisonment, so there is no escape from the dilemma unless more accurate methods are used to measure changes in the energy stores of the body. A recent development in the measurement of body density may provide this means of escape (Diethelm et al., 1977).

6.3.2. Clinical application of density measurements

The measurement of body density as an index of obesity was pioneered by Behnke et al. (1942) and developed by many investigators (Goldman and Buskirk, 1961; Siri, 1961; Durnin and Rahaman, 1967). The density of tissues has been measured (Allen et al., 1959) and the validity of the method for estimating the fat content of sheep has been confirmed by chemical analysis of their homogenised bodies (Beeston, 1965). Human fat at body temperature has a density of 0.900×10^3 kg/m^3, and a reasonable approximation for the density of the fat-free body is 1.10×10^3 kg/m^3 (Keys and Brozek, 1953). Therefore a person in whom half of his body weight was fat would have an average density of 1.000. Obviously any mixture of fat and lean will result in an average density somewhere between 1.10 and 0.90, and making the assumptions stated above it is possible to calculate percentage of fat from average body density.

The practical problem is to make a very accurate estimate of the volume of the tissues of a human subject in a manner acceptable to patients. Few patients are able and willing to immerse themselves totally but gently in water so the volume of water displaced can be accurately measured, either by displacement or from the apparent weight loss of the submerged subject. These measurements cannot be made unless the water around the subject is at rest, and in practice this means that the subject must submerge calmly and remain still under water for about 30 sec. This is perfectly easy if you understand what is needed and have confidence in the competence of the investigator, but it is not easy to induce this state of mind in all patients.

A major technical advance was that of Irsigler et al. (1975), who combined the good qualities of the usual water immersion plethysmograph with the acceptability of the gaseous system of Siri (1961): their subjects were immersed in water up to the neck, but their head was in a clear plastic cover. The volume of the airspace around the subjects head was estimated by noting the pressure change produced by withdrawing a known volume of water from the plethysmograph. However this system still has snags which affect both its acceptability and the reproducibility of the results. The general principle has been adopted, but the apparatus has been considerably modified by Diethelm et al. (1977), and the construction of the modified apparatus is shown in Fig. 6.8.

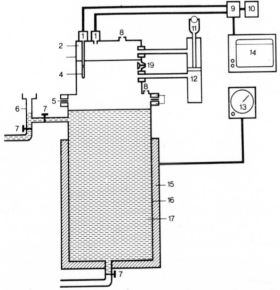

Fig. 6.8. Whole body plethysmograph based on a design by Irsigler et al. (1975) but modified by Diethelm et al. (1977). For description see text.

The features which have been copied from the design of Irsigler et al. (1975) are the vertical water tank in which the subject stands (17) and a clear plastic cover which is sealed to the tank with metal rings and a silicone rubber gasket (5). The tank is lagged (15) and the temperature of the water is recorded with an electric thermometer (13). The novel features are that the pressure changes are produced by a motor driven pump (11) and alternate between positive and negative cycles, that the pump is also connected to a reference chamber (2), and electronic pressure transducers (1) compare the pressure cycles in the space around the head of the subject with those produced in the reference chamber. Both the airspace around the subject and the reference chamber are connected to the outside air by small leaks (8) to prevent drift in the baseline pressure between the two chambers due to any change in barometric pressure or changes in volume, temperature or humidity in the air around the subject. The output of the transducers is fed to a unit which compares the signal from the two chambers (9), compares the difference with a reference voltage from a power unit (10) and displays the answer on a recorder (14).

The system is made more acceptable to patients because it is recessed into the floor and hence is easy to enter, there is a flow of air continuously around the subject's head and a microphone-loudspeaker (19) allows the subject and operator to communicate at all times. The stability and reproducibility of the system are greatly increased by using a balanced alternating system, in which unwanted changes in pressure are allowed for by comparison with the reference chamber.

It is still too early to be sure if this development will provide a reliable check on changes in body composition. Certainly it would not be adequate alone, since measurements of density involve assumptions about the composition of the lean body similar to those which limit the accuracy of estimations based on water or potassium estimations. However, the combination of a precise measurement of total body water by the method of Halliday and Miller (1977) and a measurement of density should provide a reliable estimate of body composition which does not depend much on assumed relationships of one component to another. The density of fat is fixed and known, so the density of lean tissue depends mostly on the proportion of water and bone in the fat-free body. If water is independently measured the uncertainty mainly concerns bone. Methods for estimating bone mineral have been described (Kairento and Spring, 1974; Dalen et al., 1975), but they are neither very convenient nor very accurate. It seems unlikely that changes in the mineral content of obese patients on a reducing diet would invalidate the interpretation of density measurements, but it remains to be seen if this is so.

6.3.3. The problem of the labile glycogen pool

In the model of body composition illustrated in Figs. 6.2 and 6.3 the glycogen—water pool was represented by 500 g glycogen and 1.5 kg water. This small part of the energy stores of the body is highly labile, but very difficult to measure directly. It is easy to infer its existence from the changes in weight by small degrees of energy imbalance (see Fig. 2.2) and probably it is the depletion of this glycogen pool which accounts for the rapid initial weight loss with a ketogenic diet (Yang and Van Itallie, 1976). However, it would be helpful if there was a method for measuring total body glycogen which did not involve multiple muscle biopsies (Hultman, 1967; Olsson and Saltin, 1970; Edwards, 1971).

It is fortunate that the glycogen—water pool has about the same energy value and about the same density as lean tissue, so probably fluctuations in glycogen would not invalidate estimates of the body energy stores based on measurements of water and density.

6.4. Models of "set point" and "buffer" control systems

In the previous edition of this book (Garrow, 1974b) a long section (pp. 210—224) was devoted to a discussion of different models of the control system which might regulate energy balance in man. It would be unjustifiable to rehearse these arguments again at such length, so the conclusion will be restated and then examined in the light of evidence which has become available since 1974 when the previous version was published.

The general layout of the system is shown in Fig. 6.9. Much of it

140

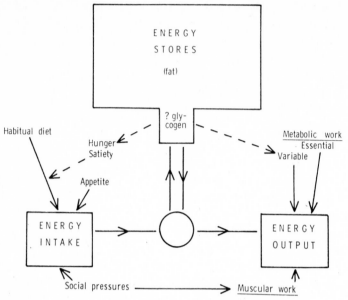

Fig. 6.9. Control system regulating energy balance in man (Garrow, 1974b).

is uncontroversial: energy stores (represented by the central rectangle) certainly consist mainly of fat with a small and variable glycogen component. It is certainly true that the size of the energy stores is determined by the balance between energy intake (the box on the left) and energy output (the box on the right). These communicate through an unlabelled circle in the middle: the common metabolic pool never closely defined but often found in such diagrams.

The controversial aspect concerns the factors which influence energy intake and output, how these factors operate and in what circumstances they arise. These have been discussed in Chapters 4 and 5.

The model in Fig. 6.9 indicates that the factors which influence energy intake are the habitual diet, modified (somewhat weakly) by the physiological signals of hunger and satiety and more strongly by appetite and social pressures. There is nothing in recent research which tends to undermine that position and quite a lot which strengthens it. The influence of habit (otherwise known as conditioning) on intake is beautifully shown by the work of Booth (1977), which shows that people will go on eating what used to be appropriate for some time after the conditions have been changed so that it is in fact inappropriate. Similarly Rozin (1976) finds that dietary conservatism is a strong influence in eating behaviour, and probably an important factor in maintaining the health and integrity of primitive communities. The fallibility of the hunger and satiety signals was already established in 1974 by the work of Wooley et al. (1972), but is confirmed by many other workers such as Pudel and Oetting (1977). The text explaining the arrow for hunger and satiety originating from that part of the energy labelled "glycogen" says: "It is easier to conceive these responses (hunger and satiety) being proportional to the amount of stored glycogen rather than the amount of fat, but further than that it would be impossible to go without unfounded speculation" (Garrow, 1974b). The foundations for this speculation are still insecure, but have received some reinforcement from the recent observations of Van Itallie et al. (1977).

The idea that appetite is an influence on intake which is powerful and unrelated to any control system is also in harmony with recent research. The Osborne—Mendel rats studied by Faust et al. (1977) find a high fat diet very palatable and readily become obese on it. My own excursion into obesity (Garrow and Stalley, 1975) was made easier by my appetite for plain chocolate digestive biscuits, to which I am very partial. Had I been restricted to milk chocolate digestive biscuits (which I do not much like) it would have been very difficult to overeat enough to gain 7 kg in 2 months. Appetite is difficult to study, since individuals vary in what they find palatable, but it is certainly a powerful influence on intake, as the work of Cabanac and Rabe (1976) confirms. "Social pressures", the last factor shown acting on food intake in Fig. 6.9, were only vaguely described in the text (Garrow, 1974b) and it is hard to define them more accurately now. The influences which affect the "restrained eaters" of Herman and Mack (1975) or the "latent obese" of Pudel and Oetting (1977) are social pressures: they arise because man is a social animal and attaches importance to his status within his society. It is hard to imagine anyone who was free from all social pressures — a complete dropout or castaway — being a restrained eater or latent obese in the terminology of these investigators. Indeed the work of Wyrwicka (1976) shows how powerful social pressures may be in the most unlikely circumstances. The protective mechanism of bait-shyness would not work unless even the most unsophisticated animals were sensitive to, and influenced by, the eating habits of other members of their species.

There seems no reason to alter the intake half (or the output half) of Fig. 6.9 in the light of recent knowledge. Methods for measuring energy expenditure have improved, but the ideas about how it is regulated have not changed much in the last 4 years: a recent review of this field (Garrow, 1978) reveals roughly the same level of ignorance as the previous attempt (Garrow, 1974b), but the situation may well improve in the next few years. At least there is no reason to retract the suggestion that energy expenditure is mainly determined by the cost of resting metabolism, and that this alters in response to overfeeding or underfeeding.

When all this is said, the chief question remains unanswered. Fig. 6.9 may be a true picture of the forces affecting energy balance, but it does not explain what *controls* it, or, in the person who becomes obese or emaciated, fails to control it.

The question in that form is unanswerable: no one has identified a switch which flicks from one position to another in certain defined conditions so as to promote positive or negative energy balance. It is naive to look for such a switch, since it probably does not exist. However, it is sensible to look for the characteristic of the system which tends to promote stability, in the way in which an economist might examine the commercial structure of a society or a particular industry to assess its economic stability.

We can identify 3 features of the system which at least tend to promote stability of energy balance. The mechanisms of hunger and satiety are imprecise, but anyone who tries to double or halve his habitual food intake will find that it is difficult to keep this up for long. Forbes (1977) shows that it is possible to predict a plateau weight for an animal if simple rules are assumed about the amount the animal can eat and the energy density of its food. Therefore even crude control of food intake will "buffer" the system against large imbalances.

The next stabilising influence is that the storage of energy involves energy expenditure: there are "banking charges" against deposits, while the cost of withdrawing energy from the stores is low. Thus overfeeding increases energy expenditure somewhat, and the resulting dietary induced thermogenesis is another factor buffering the system against large changes in energy stores (Dugdale and Payne, 1977).

The third factor is a longer-term version of the second. Large changes in body weight are associated with changes in metabolic rate, so if intake is changed from one level to another and held constant at the new level a new equilibrium will eventually be reached. It seems likely that this long-term resetting of resting metabolic rate is associated with a resetting of the rate of turnover of tissue protein (Garrow, 1974b), but there is no good evidence for or against this hypothesis.

These considerations explain to some extent the tendency of body weight to change rather slowly, but they do not explain the stability shown by individuals such as Fox (1973). To explain stability of this order it is necessary to have some feedback system correcting for drift in the "buffer" control system. The evidence indicates that in most people this feedback is conscious "when the change in body weight is no longer acceptable" (Garrow, 1974b). There may be other explanations, but it is hard to find evidence for them.

If this assessment is correct, it does not necessarily follow that obesity is a condition in which a high body weight is acceptable: this cannot be true, or nobody would complain of obesity. James and Trayhurn (1976) and Payne and Dugdale (1977) have proposed good hypotheses about the causes of obesity and the way in which there is metabolic control of body weight. If it is so, as James and Trayhurn (1976) suggest, that obese people are genetically poor at raising a thermogenic response, then the second and third stabilising factor in the control system would not buffer the system effectively, and cognitive feedback control would be placed under a greater strain and might often fail. The model of Payne and Dugdale (1977) ingeneously incorporates a differential scale of banking charges for lean and fat people and thus alters the effectiveness of the second stabilising factor, but also allows for interaction between cognitive and metabolic control systems. The essential features of these models are testable in individual obese (and latent obese) people, and it will probably turn out that some people fit better with one model, and others with another.

6.5. *Summary: the control of energy balance in man*

Primitive man may have had an automatic pilot which regulated the amount of energy he spent in gathering food and the amount of primitive food he consumed to provide tolerable regulation of energy balance during his short life-span. Modern supermarket man has no such automatic facility.

Metabolic adaptations to overfeeding and underfeeding can be demonstrated and these tend to limit weight gain or loss, but there is no evidence for a "set point" of weight in man, nor is it necessary to postulate one to explain the observed stability of body weight in most individuals. Conscious control of food intake and energy expenditure is the most probable explanation for the observed oscillations in weight about a preferred level.

No single "cause" of obesity can be identified. Statements that it is caused by (for example) inactivity cannot be proved or disproved, since the factors which influence intake (see Chapter 4) or output (see Chapter 5) are all relevant to the state of energy balance of an individual. The imbalance required to cause obesity is small compared with the range of individual variation in either intake or output of energy.

Techniques for measuring energy balance have improved greatly, and there are good hypotheses which can now be tested. It is likely that our understanding of the factors which control energy balance in man will advance rapidly in the next few years.

CHAPTER 7

The treatment of obesity

"We are unanimous in our belief that obesity is a hazard to health and a detriment to well-being. It is common enough to constitute one of the most important medical and public health problems of our time, whether we judge importance by a shorter expectation of life, increased morbidity or cost to the community in terms of both money and anxiety." Thus begins the report of a group set up to advise the authorities in this country about priorities for research (DHSS/MRC Study Group, 1976). This is good advice for governments, but it is not easy to apply to individuals. Similar statements are made by expert groups who advise governments in developing countries, but their opening paragraph may say: "We are unanimous in our belief that illiteracy is one of the major obstacles to economic development in this country", and they would probably be correct. Both obesity and illiteracy are, in general, handicaps and good governments will seek to reduce such handicaps in the populations which they serve, but when these principles are applied to individuals the results are often paradoxical. Somerset Maugham has a story about a man who was sacked from his job as a verger in a fashionable church because his employers were shocked to discover that he could not read or write. Despite this disability he became the owner of a very successful chain of tobacconist shops. In later life he was asked if he did not regret his illiteracy: surely he could have been even more successful financially if he had better schooling? He replied that on the contrary, had he been literate he would still be the verger of St. Peter's, Neville Square.

7.1. Treatment of obesity: indications and criteria

7.1.1. The disadvantages of obesity

Before considering methods of treatment for obesity it is necessary to review the disadvantages of being obese, and the likelihood that treatment will decrease these disabilities, without the cure involving greater hardship to the patient than the disease. Astwood (1962) cites a patient who thus addressed his physician in 1825: "Sir, I have followed your prescription as if my life depended upon it, and I have ascertained that during this month I have lost 3 pounds or a little more. But in order to reach this result I have been obliged to do such violence to all my tastes and all my habits − in a word I have suffered so much − that while giving you my best thanks for your kind directions, I renounce any advantages from them and throw myself for the future entirely into the hands of Providence." Although few will have expressed themselves so eloquently, there must be many patients who share these sentiments, and this is a fact which the physician must bear constantly in mind. If any doctor finds it extraordinary that his patients find it difficult to adhere strictly to a diet, even though it is plainly in their interests to do so, let him try the experiment himself. The inconvenience of consistent long-term dieting will soon become apparent.

The mortality and morbidity associated with obesity has been reviewed many times: a good recent review is that of Bray (1976). It is, in my view, unfortunate that the debate about the importance of obesity as a risk to health tends to focus on the relative chances of fat or thin men aged 50 dying prematurely from a heart attack. Epidemiologists who design trials want results they can analyse: Keys et al. (1972) knew that if they set up a prospective study of 2442 U.S. railwaymen, 2439 men in northern Europe and 6519 in southern Europe, and followed them for 5 years, it would involve a great deal of work. They selected men aged 40−59 years at entry to the study, and in this massive series had 163 cases of death or definite myocardial infarction. If they had chosen men aged 20−39 at entry they would have had just as much work and had far fewer deaths to analyse, so middle-aged men tend to attract the attention of epidemiologists (who are themselves often middle-aged men). The answer obtained by Keys et al. (1972) was that if a skinfold thickness (triceps + subscapular) of 36 mm was used to differentiate obese from lean, then 20.5% of all the men (and 52.3% of the American railwaymen) were obese. Among the obese men 2.67% had heart attacks in the 5 years of the study, and 1.60% of the lean man. However, if age, blood pressure, serum cholesterol and smoking were also taken into account then obesity made no independent contribution to future coronary heart disease. Similar results have recently been published by Pelkonen et al. (1977), who showed that among Finns aged 50–53 the chance of death from heart disease was associated with overweight in those who also had raised cholesterol (>7.8 mmoles/l) or triglycerides (>1.70 mmoles/l), but those with normal blood lipids showed no relationship between obesity and cardiovascular death.

If we accept that a man of 50 is not at significantly greater risk of a coronary thrombosis if he is overweight unless he also has raised blood lipids, we now need to know if his hyperlipidaemia is in turn related to his body fat. Weinsier et al. (1976) studied 1483 American aircrew aged 17–64 and found a statistically significant relationship between body fat and blood pressure, cholesterol and triglycerides ($P < 0.01$) but commented that it was only of small magnitude. However, if you are overweight, have high blood lipids and want to avoid coronary heart disease, probably the most constructive step you can take is to reduce weight (Leelartheapin et al., 1974).

When we consider younger age groups the association between overweight and early death becomes much clearer. The data in Table 7.1 are taken from a study by Blair and Haines (1966) on 5408 policies issued at standard rates by the Provident Mutual insurance company. All policy holders had passed a medical examination. The figures in the table show the percentage of average mortality observed by age at issue, deviation from standard weight and duration of the policy. Where less than 25 deaths occurred in an age/weight/policy year group no value is given.

It is evident from the life insurance figures (of which Table 7.1 shows a sample) that overweight shortens life more in the young than in the middle-aged. Professional epidemiologists are sceptical of conclusions based on insurance statistics, since the subjects are not a random sample of the population, but are self-selected. It might be that

148

TABLE 7.1

PERCENTAGE OF AVERAGE MORTALITY IN MEN WHO PASSED A MEDI-
CAL EXAMINATION FOR LIFE INSURANCE, DIVIDED BY AGE AT
EXAMINATION, DEVIATION FROM STANDARD WEIGHT, AND DURA-
TION OF POLICY AT DEATH

Dashes indicate less than 25 deaths in that age/weight/policy year group (data of
Blair and Haines, 1966).

Age at issue (years)	Deviation from standard weight	Policy years				All policies
		16−20	21−25	26−30	31−34	
15−34	−23 lb or more	102	78	80	95	86
	−22 to −8 lb	77	76	91	98	86
	−7 to +7 lb	82	107	108	108	103
	+8 to +22 lb	166	131	115	94	125
	+23 lb or more	137	184	143	−	146
35−49	−23 lb or more	67	84	86	72	80
	−22 to −8 lb	79	83	77	84	80
	−7 to +7 lb	104	91	105	86	99
	+8 to +22 lb	116	117	108	119	115
	+23 lb or more	119	134	132	169	130
50−65	−23 lb or more	−	−	120	−	95
	−22 to −8 lb	97	108	102	−	100
	−7 to +7 lb	98	87	81	88	90
	+8 to +22 lb	109	102	113	−	108
	+23 lb or more	107	125	122	−	118

fat people who get a touch of angina fear death, and rush off to
become insured, thus biassing the sample. This is indeed possible,
but, if this is true, it is all the more remarkable that overweight people who have been refused insurance at normal premiums enjoy normal life expectancy if they reduce their weight to the "desirable
range". This conclusion is based on a review of 2300 people by
Dublin (1953) who comments: "A test of this kind is about as objective as one could ask."

So far I have avoided the difficult task of defining obesity. It is
easy to generate platitudinous statements like: "Obesity is a condition caused by an excessive amount of adipose tissue", which,
although true, are practically useless unless you also explain how to
measure the amount of fat in a person and decide if it is excessive. In

marginal cases this is impossible to do. In the slightly overweight it can be argued that it is important to distinguish between adiposity and muscularity (Parnell, 1977), but in the grossly overweight this problem does not arise. For practical clinical purposes it is convenient to take the range of "desirable weight" from life insurance experience, from the lower end of the small frame to the upper end of the large frame (since frame size is undefined), and accept that people above this range are obese. This simple guide is shown in Fig. 7.1 (Garrow, 1974b).

By this standard some athletes will be wrongly classified as obese, and some old people who have excessive body fat will appear in the "desirable range". This is a small price to pay for the simplicity of the classification, since athletes and old people are fairly easy to recognise, and the values can be interpreted accordingly. The relationship of body fat to relative weight was studied by Lesser et al. (1971); their results are shown in Fig. 7.2. For young men and women criteria of overweight (more than 110% relative body weight) and excess fat (more than 22% fat for men and 28% for women) agree fairly well, but in the older age groups the relationship breaks down. Again,

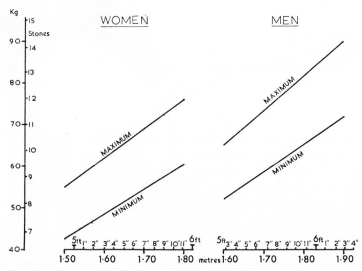

Fig. 7.1. Range of desirable weight for height in men and women wearing indoor clothing.

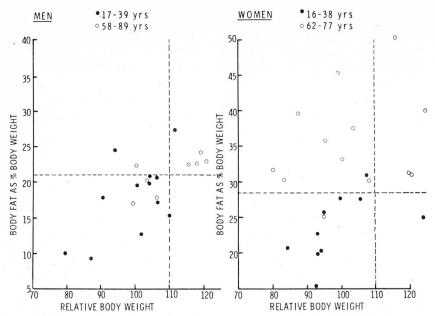

Fig. 7.2. Relationship of relative body weight to percentage body fat in young and old men and women (data of Lesser et al., 1971).

from a clinical viewpoint this does not matter much, since old people who are obese are difficult to treat and benefit relatively little from weight reduction even if it is achieved.

It may be objected that the range of desirable weight given in Fig. 7.1 is too wide: for a man 1.7 m tall it stretches from 58 to 74 kg, which in terms of body mass index (W/H^2) is 20–25.6. However, even at the upper end of the range the effect on mortality is small: indeed, in a small series from the Chicago Peoples Gas Company, Dyer et al. (1975) found a minimum mortality associated with a body mass index of 23.6–25.6. Mortality with an index above 31 is very high (Sorensen and Sonne-Holm, 1977).

It is difficult to obtain reliable information about the morbidity associated with overweight. Rimm et al. (1975) analysed 73,522 questionnaires from women who were members of the slimming club TOPS. They were asked questions of the form: "Has a doctor ever said you had . . .?" for a variety of diseases, so the results tell us what overweight women think they were told. However, when the answers are analysed by degree of overweight, going from the lowest group at only 10.1% overweight to the highest at 85.3% overweight, trends in reported diagnosis are evident. The most overweight women in the 30—39-year age range (in which there were most replies) reported 4.8% with a diagnosis of diabetes, 47.1% with high blood pressure and 21.8% with gall bladder disease, compared with 1.2% diabetes, 13.6% high blood pressure and 7.2% gall bladder disease in women of the same age in the least overweight group. The most overweight women did not consistently overreport all diagnoses: their claims to a diagnosis of heart disease, anaemia and jaundice do not show the same high ratios, and the implication that increasing overweight is associated with increasing prevalence of diabetes, hypertension and gall bladder disease is confirmed by the insurance companies' experience (Donald, 1973). Blitzer (1976) found from a survey of 56,111 members of TOPS clubs that there was in general no association between overweight and cancer, but that those who were very obese teenagers had an increased risk (by a factor 1.62) of endometrial cancer. Osteoarthritis of the knees is very common in overweight women over the age of 50 (Leach et al., 1973) and is greatly helped by weight reduction (Dixon and Henderson, 1973). However, this association has not been found in men (Lawrence, 1975). A clinic in California in which 261 people came for a free medical evaluation of their obesity (Bray et al., 1976b) found that 25% had raised triglycerides, 11% raised cholesterol and 7% abnormal uric acid or alkaline phosphatase in serum. Among the women 27% had menstrual abnormalities, but this does not necessarily reflect the prevalence in obese women generally.

The obese patient certainly causes problems for the obstetrician, surgeon and anaesthetist. Peckham and Christiansen (1971) analysed the obstetric records of 3939 women in California: they compared the performance of the 10% of women whose pre-pregnancy weight was lightest, average or heaviest at each height range. Their "light" group was near the lower limit of the range of desirable weight shown in Fig. 7.1, the "average" group was in the upper half of that range, and the "heavy" group was above the upper limit of the range. Toxaemia and hypertension increased with increasing weight grouping: 0.3%, 1.5% and 7.9% for toxaemia, and 2.0%, 2.6% and 6.4% for hypertension. In primipara labour was longest in the heavy group by 2 h, but not in multipara. The relationship of maternal to fetal obesity is discussed in Section 7.9. Certainly obesity in pregnancy increases the risks both to the mother and the child (Efiong, 1975; Maeder et al., 1975).

The pulmonary function of obese patients is poor: Bae et al. (1976) found that 10 obese patients weighing on average 154 kg had a smaller functional lung capacity than normal men of the same age who weighed on average 64 kg, so the pulmonary reserve is very small. Bray (1976) reports similar impairment of lung function in obese patients. With anaesthesia the situation becomes much worse (Fisher et al., 1975), it is difficult to maintain adequate oxygenation (Hedenstierna and Santesson, 1976) especially if the patient is tilted head down (Paul et al., 1976; Vaughan and Wise, 1976), the adipose mass makes it difficult to maintain the appropriate concentration of anaesthetic gas (Saraiva et al., 1977) and the obese patient is more liable to aspirate gastric juice (Vaughan et al., 1975). Meanwhile the surgeon has problems getting into the abdominal cavity, finding what he is looking for and closing the wound satisfactorily: special techniques have been devised to cope with obese surgical patients (Loffer and Pent, 1976; Morrow et al., 1977).

7.1.2. Indications for treatment: who treats whom?

From the previous section it appears that the individuals who are most likely to suffer from obesity are the young, the very obese and those about to undergo surgery. By losing weight they are likely to reduce their chance of developing diabetes, hypertension, gall bladder disease and osteoarthritis of weight-bearing joints. They will probably increase their expectation of life, improve exercise tolerance and certainly fare better if they require surgery. Men with angina may be helped with weight loss, but not necessarily so (Sharma et al., 1974). Obese patients often expect that weight loss will improve their social life: sometimes this is so, but not always, and it may be that some are happier when fat (Crisp and McGuiness, 1976).

This assessment of what is to be gained by weight loss is evidently not shared by all obese patients, nor their doctors. The Consumers' Association in the U.K. asked its members who had experience of trying to lose weight to fill in a questionnaire and received 2333 replies. Of these 1362 people (1117 women and 245 men) had received advice from their family doctor; roughly half had consulted their doctor specifically about their weight, and the others had consulted him about something else but had been given advice about losing weight (Ashwell, 1973). Only 28% of women and 27% of men were asked to return regularly to the doctor to check on progress (they were almost all N.H.S. patients, so no charge was involved in such a return visit) and 9% of women and 7% of men were told not to worry about their weight. The picture which emerges is that about half the people answering the questionnaire had not had medical advice on weight loss, and of those who had advice from the doctor only half had actively sought it and some of these had been discouraged from weight loss. It may well be that these were teenage girls with anorectic tendencies who should indeed have been discouraged from weight loss. At least it is plain that only a minority of people in the survey were being treated at all by their doctors, and since only 28% were asked to come back the level of enthusiasm shown by the doctors cannot have been high.

Most people who seriously want to lose weight and do not get (or expect) much help from their family doctor will try a slimming club. There are 3 nationwide clubs in the U.K.: Weight Watchers, Slimming Magazine Club and Silhouette Slimming Club, and innumerable small local clubs, some of which are based on sound principles and some of which are quite incompetent. A survey of a random sample of the membership of the 3 national clubs in the U.K. was answered by 341 women one year after enrolling in the club: this is a 56.8% response to the 600 questionnaires sent out, and the response rate was similar for all the clubs (Ashwell and Garrow, 1975). The results were also generally similar: on average members attended for about 6 months and lost about 11 kg. Among the women who answered the questionnaire there were 136 who had lost at least 6.35 kg while attending the club, but had ceased attending club meetings. In order to find out the permanence of their weight loss a second letter was sent to these women, of whom 92 (68%) replied. Most of them (63%) had regained some of the weight they had lost while attending the club, 16.3% had regained it all and 7.6% were above the weight at which they joined the club. However, 10.9% said they had maintained their weight loss and 2.2% had lost even more weight since leaving the club. A fuller and more recent review of the characteristics of clubs in several countries by Ashwell (1978a) shows a similar picture.

So what responsibility has the medical profession to treat obese patients? According to some authors, very little. Young (1963), addressing the American Medical Association in Atlantic City, advises against indiscriminate help to any obese patient. "Only the patient for whom there is some likelihood of success, and for whom undesirable sequellae are unlikely, should be encouraged to undertake weight reduction." Those likely to succeed can be identified by their stable personality, high motivation, late onset of obesity and absence of any previous unsuccessful attempt at weight loss! Similar sentiments guide Shearer and Kiely (1977) who describe "new techniques for office management of obesity." It transpires that these are not techniques to help the *patient,* but a computer programme to help the doctor to identify "non-responders", that is, patients who will fail to lose weight "and were therefore not worth spending additional time on." So efficient is this programme that by the time they had discarded non-responders they had only 16 patients left at 16 weeks, having started with 54.

This policy will greatly increase the apparent success rate among doctors treating obesity, but the highly motivated patients with stable personality would probably have done very well at a slimming club, and it is not clear who is supposed to help the early-onset obese who *have* previously tried, and failed, to lose weight. If the advice of Young (1963) is applied generally in medicine, doctors will insist on treating only infectious diseases caused by an organism which is sensitive to a convenient antibiotic and will not think it worth spending additional time on infarcts, chronic arthritis, or any degenerative or terminal disease, since there is so little chance of success, and undesirable sequellae are all too likely.

7.1.3. Criteria for success in treatment
Innumerable pages suggesting some new line of treatment for obes-

ity open with a statement to the effect: "Since conventional dietary management of obesity almost always fails . . ." and there follows a reference either to the original paper of Stunkard and McLaren-Hume (1959) or to some more recent paper which itself quotes the same source (e.g. Bray, 1970b; Stunkard, 1972). To set the record straight, Stunkard and McLaren-Hume (1959) reviewed all the publications available at that time in which both weight loss and drop-out rate were recorded. Only outpatient treatment was considered, since "inpatient treatment, with its far greater control over food intake, does not present the same problems." They found 8 reports between 1931 and 1958, and set as a criterion of "success" a weight loss of 20 lb, which was "indeed a small weight loss for the grossly overweight persons who are the subjects of these reports." They conclude that only 25% were able to lose as much as 20 lb and only 5% lost 40 lb, and since the reports were written by experts in the field "It is probable that their results, poor as they seem, are nevertheless better than those obtained by the average physician."

This may well be true, but the average physician is probably not really trying: perhaps people like Stunkard and Young have persuaded him he ought not to try. Non-average physicians who *do* try do better: for example Craddock (1977) reports that 43 patients (28.7% of a series in general practice) lost 20 lb, and 29 (19.3%) maintained this loss for at least 10 years. Among those who replied to the slimming club survey (Ashwell and Garrow, 1975), 54.2% lost between 14 and 42 lb and 6.3% lost more than 42 lb. However, these results are not achieved without effort by the patient and sensible advice and encouragement from someone else, either a doctor, or slimming club leader, or perhaps a friend or relative. Hospital doctors do better because, as Stunkard says, control of food intake is easier with inpatients. The weight loss achieved by obese patients is very closely related to the amount of trouble which their advisers are prepared to take, a fact which is clearly shown in the survey by Ashwell (1973).

The problem is to define the amount of effort which doctor and patient can reasonably be expected to contribute, and the "success" which this effort is likely to bring. Weight loss is not a very good criterion of success: it is easy to measure and analyse, which is why Stunkard uses it, but it is not true that the series they reviewed consisted of "grossly overweight persons" for whom "20 lb is indeed a small weight loss": some patients were only 3% overweight and some were treated for only 3 weeks, so these can hardly have needed or expected to lose 20 lb, and still less 40 lb. In the treatment of obesity, as in the treatment of other diseases, "success" is achieving what was hoped for at the start of treatment — usually the relief of some pain or disability. The respects in which weight loss is likely to improve well-being are listed at the beginning of Section 7.2. The fat ugly embarrassed girl who hopes weight loss will bring social success, and who after losing 20 kg is a thin ugly embarrassed girl with no friends is a "failure" so far as treatment is concerned, while the woman with osteoarthritic knees who is enabled to climb the stairs in her home after losing 8 kg is a "success". This is not academic hair-splitting: it is an important practical point to be kept in mind when, for example, trying to compare the "success" of total starvation or of exercise in the treatment of obesity. A few days of starvation will achieve as much weight loss as weeks of exercise, but this is not a sound basis on which to compare their success rate.

It is probably fair to say that the chances of "success" in treating an obese patient are similar to the chances of "success" in teaching an Englishman to speak German. To paraphrase the splendid rhetoric of Stunkard (1972) on the ineffectiveness of such efforts we might say: "Most Englishmen learning German give up after a year or two at school. Of those who persist most never speak fluent German. Of those who do achieve fluency, most do not keep it up." Few people would argue from this evidence that it is impossible to learn German, since there are currently some 80 million German-speaking people, and people (even Englishmen) who really need to learn German to earn a living often do so. Similarly, leaders of slimming groups who have lost weight and would be sacked if they regained it do remarkably well (Bender and Bender, 1976). Of course there are individual differences in the facility with which people lose weight or learn foreign languages, and in the amount of weight loss (or language proficiency) they need to achieve. However, it is as absurd to say "obesity is an incurable disease" (Sash, 1977) as to claim that German is an unlearnable language. There are currently diseases (like multiple sclerosis) for which I know no treatment worth troubling the patient with, and it is a cruel deception in such circumstances to pretend that the medical profession can offer a cure. Obesity is in quite a different class of disease, and it seems an equally cruel deception to tell a fat person who wants, and needs, to lose weight that this is impossible. What the patient needs is a reasonable estimate of cost-effectiveness: what can they expect to lose, in how long, by what means, and if they do, what can they expect to gain, and is it worth it? Doctors are often asked for such cost-effectiveness advice: should the man with angina give up golf? should the bronchitic change to a lower-paid but easier job in better working conditions? should the mother of two handicapped children try to have another child?

There is no correct answer to these questions, but the purpose of this book is to assemble the information about the causes, effects and treatment of obesity so the doctor can make an informed estimate about which obese patients he can help.

An interesting report by Binnie (1977) records the excess weight and weight change in 43 patients treated in a single-handed rural practice in the north of England with about 1200 patients. The treatment of obesity was not given special importance in this practice, but what the author describes modestly as "average general practice management". In fact it was probably better than average: it was his policy to weigh patients, and those overweight were advised to follow the Marriott diet (low carbohydrate) as recommended by Craddock (1973). They were asked to return in 4 weeks, and if they had lost weight they were encouraged to persevere with the diet, but if not various anorectic drugs were tried. The results of this eminently reasonable policy are shown in Fig. 7.3. Binnie (1977) classifies the 5 patients shown by open circles as successes, since after 10 years they were within 10% of an "ideal weight" standard, somewhat stricter than that shown in Fig. 7.1. The broken line shows the perfect result in which weight loss would exactly equal the original excess weight: it is obvious that most of the results are far from perfect. But surely the woman who "after deciding to forgo medication and keep to her own regime of eating less lost 21 kg (47 lb), and although still 45% overweight is satisfied with her present, much improved outline" is also a great success?

158

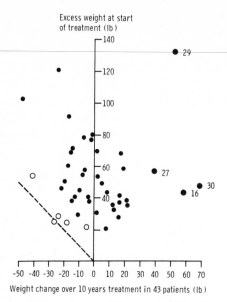

Fig. 7.3. Excess weight and weight change in 43 patients treated in general practice (data of Binnie, 1977). Those rated "successes" by Binnie are shown as open circles.

In 4 patients in Fig. 7.3 the situation is clearly disastrous, since 10 years ago they were more than 40 lb overweight and during the last 10 years they have not lost, but gained, at least as much again. The ages of these patients are shown in Fig. 7.3: they are less than 30 years old and if present trends continue their prognosis is very poor. By the criteria of Young (1963), Shearer and Keily (1977), Gray and Kallenbach (1939), Goldrick et al. (1973) and many others these are clearly non-responders who do not deserve further attention, but before accepting this policy it would be well to know *why* they were non-responders. Were they aware of the dangers of the course they were following, and happy to accept the consequences? It is more likely that they believe that they have an incurable disease, so there is no point in fighting it: after all no less an authority than Astwood (1962) said: "I wish to propose that obesity is an inherited disorder and due to a genetically determined effect in an enzyme: in other words that people who are fat are born fat, and nothing much can be done about it." Perhaps this is so of some people, but not of most. The genetic component of obesity is discussed by Garrow (1976). However, a patient aged 29 who was 133 lb overweight at age 19, and who now weighs 290 lb (132 kg) with a height of 59 in. (1.5 m), clearly needs more help than she will get from a Marriott diet. No doubt she observes that her friends and relations can eat far more than she does without gaining weight, and the slimming pills which work so well for others have little effect on her weight, so it would not be surprising if she has given up hope.

In Victorian times it was customary to give up hope with many diseases which we would now investigate, diagnose and treat. I think that all the patients more than 60 lb (27 kg) overweight in Fig. 7.3 have a disease sufficiently serious to justify similar investigation, and certainly the young patients who are currently gaining weight. Methods for estimating the energy expenditure of these patients are described in Chapter 3, factors affecting energy expenditure are discussed in Chapter 5, and the range of energy expenditure which may be found is indicated in the summary to that chapter. Before considering what treatment is appropriate for patients in whom a large energy deficit is required, it is helpful to know their energy output, since it is then possible to make a reasonable calculation of the weight loss to be expected on a given energy intake.

7.1.4. Summary: when to try hard, when to give up

Anyone above the weight-for-height range in Fig. 7.1, unless they are unusually muscular, would do well to lose weight. The younger, and the more overweight, the more they stand to gain from weight loss. Such people will probably have tried to lose weight with advice from a magazine or slimming club before asking medical advice. Often this advice is poor or has been misunderstood, or the individual thinks the weight loss achieved is not worth the effort involved, or cannot understand why others lose more weight on the same diet.

The first step in rational treatment of such a patient is to try to assess the probable benefit to the patient of weight loss in the short term (not losing job as air hostess) or long term (not getting diabetes). If the benefit is negligible, as for people already in the normal range of weight, say so.

If the benefit to the patient is substantial it is important that the patient realises this, since achieving the weight loss is going to require considerable effort from the patient. If the patient is prepared to try hard, so should the doctor. Anything less than a monthly review of progress represents too little effort on both sides, so no doctor can treat more patients than he can afford to see monthly. Priority should go to the youngest and most overweight. Four pounds (2 kg) per month is a just-good-enough rate of weight loss, some patients will maintain higher rates, but not the 6 kg/month or more which many patients expect (Ford et al., 1977).

If a substantially overweight patient fails to maintain a rate of 2 kg/month despite (apparently) trying to follow dietary advice, a critical situation arises in which the doctor may inadvertently do serious harm. It is essential that the reason for failure should be established and not guessed. If the patient is told that it is fluid retention, or some metabolic defect, which makes weight loss impossible on a normal reducing diet, and this is *not* true, that patient has been made refractory to all future treatment. If it *is* true, the defect should be identified by the techniques described in this book and the appropriate treatment given.

If, having had a fair statement of the prognosis, the patient is not prepared to contribute at least a half-share of the necessary effort, the doctor should give up. This part of the plan is easy to follow: it is more difficult to ensure that the effort the patient is being asked to make is the right one.

7.2. Dietary treatment of obesity

Virtually all treatments of obesity which are effective are dietary treatments. The anorectic drugs, gut bypass operations and stereotactic surgery aim to reduce food intake and hence promote a negative energy balance. This section is concerned with treatments in which reliance is placed entirely on persuading the patient to alter his dietary habits, since in general this is the treatment of first choice. Much research has been done to try to predict which patients will respond favourably to such advice, or how it should be most compellingly presented (Ley et al., 1974; Rodin et al., 1977a), but without much success.

There is no evidence that obese people in general eat more than non-obese (Ries, 1973), although some of them do. Therefore the object of dietary advice is not to persuade obese patients to eat normally (since many of them do that anyway) but to eat less than they require, so as to burn their excess fat stores.

7.2.1. Total starvation

The most effective way to cause a negative energy balance is to cut off the energy intake from food completely, but total starvation in man causes complex metabolic and endocrine adaptations, not all of which are favourable. For reviews of this topic by experts see Cahill (1970) and Palmblad et al. (1977). To assess the usefulness of starvation in the treatment of obesity it is necessary to consider the practical difficulties of persuading patients to abstain totally from food, or any but acaloric drinks, the composition of the weight loss which is achieved and the dangers of the procedure.

About 10 years ago there was a vogue for intermittent starvation (Bloom, 1959; Duncan et al., 1962, 1963). The idea was that a few days of starvation produced a rapid weight loss, and the ketosis associated with starvation inhibited hunger, then a few days on a reducing diet stabilised the situation, and a further brief spell of starvation achieved further weight loss, and so on. However, the anorexia produced by brief starvation is not evident on objective testing (Silverstone et al., 1966) and the long-term results of this policy are worse than those who had a conventional low energy diet (Harrison and Harden, 1966; Maagøe and Mogensen, 1970). Intermittent starvation therefore seems useless and will not be discussed further.

To carry the clinical responsibility for patients who are totally starving is quite a burden: things go wrong even in fit young men under close observation (Kjellberg et al., 1977), and it is folly to contemplate long-term starvation as an outpatient procedure. The dangers to look out for are reviewed by Drenick (1976) and include liver damage, vitamin deficiencies, electrolyte depletion and disturbance of acid-base regulation, increase in uric acid excretion which may

TABLE 7.2

SUMMARY OF THE WEIGHT LOSS ACHIEVED BY TOTAL STARVATION IN GROSSLY OBESE PATIENTS

Author	Date	Number of cases	Duration of fast (days)		Weight loss (kg)		Mean (kg/day)
			Mean	Range	Mean	Range	
Drenick et al.	1964	11	42	(12–117)	17	(8.2–52.6)	0.41
Thomson et al.	1966	13	89	(25–249)	19	(3.6–44)	0.21
Munro et al.	1970	25	83	(4–196)	28	(3.1–59.0)	0.34
Rooth and Carlström	1970	20	47	(14–110)	18.3	(7.2–31.1)	0.39
Runcie and Thomson	1970	18	121	(69–249)	47	(20.4–64.9)	0.39
Drenick	1976	137	56	(31–124)	30	(13–78)	0.54

precipitate gout and a major loss of lean tissue. These can only be observed and controlled in inpatients, so starvation is an expensive method of treating obesity, which involves "a large investment of time, money and medical manpower" (Drenick, 1976) and a risk of sudden death (Norbury, 1964; Spencer, 1968; Garnett et al., 1969).

The rate of weight loss achieved by supervised total starvation is very high initially and decreases with time. Runcie and Hilditch (1974) review the pattern of weight loss in 58 women and 18 men who initially weighed 104 ± 18 kg and 123 ± 29 kg, respectively. Their average weight loss during the first 14 days of starvation was 7.7 ± 1.7 kg and 10.2 ± 1.8 kg for women and men respectively, but between 15 and 22 days of fasting this had decreased to 2.17 ± 0.9 and 3.02 ± 0.8 kg, and between 25 and 30 days it had become 2.18 ± 0.8 and 2.84 ± 0.7 kg. The total weight loss achieved by prolonged starvation is reported in several papers which are summarized in Table 7.2.

The nature of the tissue lost to achieve the impressive weight loss shown in Table 7.2 has been investigated by several authors. In the early stages of a fast about 10–14 g of nitrogen appear in the urine daily, representing catabolism of about 75 g of body protein (Drenick, 1976): insulin concentration falls, glucagon rises and there is a flood of amino acids out of muscle (Pozefsky et al., 1976). The peak nitrogen loss is about the third day of the fast (Göschke et al., 1975), it decreases to about 3–4 g/day by the end of the first month and thereafter declines very little for the duration of the fast.

The long-term results of prolonged fasting are also poor (Innes et al., 1974) since weight is usually rapidly regained. The search is therefore on for ways in which fasting can be modified so as to retain the advantage of rapid weight loss, but avoid the dangers and in particular the loss of lean tissue.

7.2.2. Protein-sparing modified fasts

The literature concerning nitrogen balance and energy intake in normal subjects was reviewed by Calloway and Spector (1954), who concluded that subjects in negative energy balance were also in negative nitrogen balance. On intakes down to about 800 kcal (3.4 MJ) daily loss of lean tissue increased to about 20 g protein daily, but below that level energy deficits were associated with higher rates of loss of lean tissue, so cutting the energy intake from 800 kcal to zero increased protein loss from about 20 g daily to about 75 g daily. However, in the last 20 years there have been many claims that in special circumstances the general relationship between energy deficit and protein loss can be broken: specifically that very high protein intakes, with no other energy source, could promote nitrogen balance when the total energy intake was far below the threshold value of about 800 kcal. Much of this work was initiated by observations on severely ill patients who were maintained by parenteral nutrition, since it was easy to perform nitrogen balance on a patient whose protein intake could be calculated from the bottles of amino acid infused and whose urine was easy to collect and analyse.

A recent review on protein—energy relationships in parenteral nutrition by Jeejeebhoy (1976) states that nitrogen balance is linearly related to protein input at any given level of added non-protein energy source, and that it made little difference if the non-protein energy came from glucose or fat. Thus if protein is the sole energy source and given at the rate of 0.5 g protein/kg ideal body weight/day, the patient would be losing about 6 g nitrogen/day, but if the rate of amino acid infusion was raised to 2 g/kg/day (equivalent to 140 g protein daily for a man of 70 kg) a positive nitrogen balance of about 2 g/day could be achieved. If 15 g glucose/kg/day was added to the infusion, nitrogen balance could be achieved at much lower protein inputs: 0.5 g/kg/day would achieve nitrogen equilibrium, and 2 g/kg/day a positive balance of 6 g nitrogen/day.

The observation that 15 g glucose plus 0.5 g protein/kg/day could promote nitrogen equilibrium is of no great importance to those concerned with the treatment of obesity, since a 70-kg man who received 4340 kcal (18 MJ) daily would not lose weight. However, nitrogen equilibrium on 140 g protein as a sole energy source sounds most attractive, for this is a diet with only 560 kcal (2.3 MJ) daily on which weight loss would be rapid but lean tissue would be preserved. The biochemical basis for "protein-sparing therapy" in obesity has been suggested by Flatt and Blackburn (1974). Insulin inhibits lipolysis, and a glucose load stimulates a greater release of insulin than an isocaloric amount of protein. Thus starvation ketosis may be a valuable factor in preserving body protein during fasting, and if protein can be given in the diet without stopping the ketosis, and without stimulating much insulin secretion, the body will meet its energy deficit by burning fat rather than protein. However, when the application of this general principle is examined in detail there is considerable dissent about the optimum amount of protein to give to obtain the best "protein-sparing" effect.

There is no doubt that any energy source — protein, carbohydrate or fat — will spare protein in a previously starving patient, and the main difficulty in comparing the efficacy of different nutrients in this respect is that the amount of protein sparing will depend on the previous diet. For example, Bolinger et al. (1966) compared the effect of 40 g cooked egg white with total starvation and showed that during starvation his subject lost on average 7.34 g nitrogen daily, but with the addition of 40 g protein this was reduced to 2.38 g nitrogen daily. When the protein intake was increased to 60–80 g daily nitrogen balance became positive, but ketosis and anorexia disappeared. He concluded that about 40 g protein had an optimum effect. Also in that study (but seldom quoted) is evidence that the subjects who were on 20 g fat daily (roughly equal to 40 g protein as an energy source) lost 2.88 g nitrogen daily, which is not very different from the 2.38 g on the protein supplement. Apfelbaum (1976) advocates 55 g protein in the form of casein, with which he reports nitrogen equilibrium established over the first 3 weeks of treatment.

A series of papers from the group at Massachusetts Institute of Technology claims to demonstrate nitrogen balance in patients fed on protein only, but it is very difficult to convince oneself of the validity of these claims. Blackburn et al. (1975) and Bistrian et al. (1975, 1977b) describe, to 3 significant figures, nitrogen balance measurements on patients who were fed lean beef. Bistrian et al. (1975) say that urine creatinine, urea and total nitrogen were measured, but do not give results for creatinine or urea, nor do they say how the urine was collected and preserved. In ketotic patients a large proportion of the nitrogen in urine appears as ammonia, so it is essential that the urine is acidified, or the ammonia escapes and apparent nitrogen balance becomes positive! It is stranger still that they do not explain how they measured nitrogen intake. Bistrian et al. (1977b) explain that the "nitrogen content of meat protein was determined from standard tables" and quote a positive balance of about 2 g nitrogen daily in patients who were eating 86 g of meat protein. The difficulties of measuring food intake were elaborated in Section 3.1 of this book, and a fairly charitable view of the metabolic balance procedures described by Bistrian et al. (1977b) is that they were open to errors which make the results impossible to interpret: if the nitrogen content of the meat was overestimated, or if some of the meat offered was not eaten, or if ammonia was lost from the urine (each of which is quite likely), the apparent positive nitrogen balance may well be an artefact.

The study by Bistrian et al. (1977a) uses egg protein as a diet to provide 1.5 g protein/kg ideal body weight. The ideal body weight of their subjects is not given, but the diet must have provided about 80 g protein. On this regimen nitrogen balance was not attained in 3 weeks. On the available evidence, therefore, the value of pure protein diets in preserving lean tissue has yet to be established. The ketosis which they cause makes it easier to tell if the patient is keeping to the diet (Biron et al., 1977), but is not evidence of nitrogen balance.

The effects of low energy diets which are not specifically intended to suppress insulin secretion and promote ketosis have been investigated by Jourdan et al. (1974), Genuth et al. (1974) and Howard and Baird (1977). The study by Jourdan et al. (1974) was performed under tightly controlled conditions and compared 3 levels of protein intake and 3 levels of energy intake in 6 obese women. The protocol lasted 63 days, and during the last period of 12 days the subjects were less than 1 g nitrogen in negative balance on a diet supplying about 700 kcal (3 MJ) and 20 g protein. This seems remarkable in view of the generalisation of Calloway and Spector (1954) that an intake of about 700 kcal should be associated with a loss of about 20 g protein, or 3 g nitrogen daily. The explanation is that there is a general tendency for nitrogen balance to improve with time during any low energy regimen (this was described even with total starvation in Section 7.2.1), so the protein-sparing value of a diet must always be examined in the light of the previous protocol.

The policy of Genuth et al. (1974) was to admit obese patients to hospital for a period of investigation and fasting for about one week, and then to discharge them on 75 g/day of casein and glucose: in some patients this was 30 g casein and 45 g glucose, and in others 45 g casein and 30 g glucose. No formal nitrogen balance studies were done, but this "outpatient semi-starvation" regimen was tolerated by 45 out of 75 patients for 8–50 weeks, with an average weight loss of 32 kg for women and 41 kg for men. Patients were reported to engage in normal activities and no serious disabilities were encountered. Baird et al. (1974) and Howard and Baird (1977) also used a mixture of protein and carbohydrate to provide about 250 kcal (1 MJ) daily. Rates of weight loss and drop-out rates were similar to the series of Genuth et al. (1974), but Howard and Baird (1977) also report hunger ratings and estimates of nitrogen balance in their patients. A diet with 25 g protein from egg albumen and 40 g carbohydrate daily was associated with little ketosis, not much hunger, probably nearly nitrogen balance and rapid weight loss.

It will be evident from this brief review of "protein-sparing modified fasts" that many variations have been tried, and virtually every statement on the subject is contradicted by some other investigator. According to Flatt and Blackburn (1974) the addition of carbohydrate to a marginal protein intake should increase loss of body protein, but Jeejeebhoy (1976) and Howard and Baird (1977) report the reverse. It is not clear if ketosis spares protein or reduces hunger: the observations of Silverstone et al. (1966) suggest that ketotic patients are hungry, Howard and Baird (1977) say their mildly ketotic patients were not hungry, yet it is claimed by Bolinger et al. (1966) that freedom from hunger was one of the benefits of ketosis.

Some of these contradictions may be reconciled by reference to Fig. 7.4, which shows the weight loss and nitrogen excretion of a female patient who was totally starved for 50 days and given 15 g of glucose daily from day 50 to 60, and 45 g glucose daily from day 61 to 70. Throughout the 10-week study period she had no dietary protein, but the usual vitamin and mineral supplements, and unlimited acaloric fluids. Daily determinations of total urine nitrogen were performed by the Kjeldahl procedure, as well as measurements of other nitrogenous compounds in urine, in connection with a study of protein metabolism (Halliday et al., unpublished). The curve of weight loss shows the usual rapid phase for about 5 days, followed by a very constant rate of loss of 250 g/day during the next 45 days of total starvation. Total nitrogen excretion increased to nearly 10 g/day towards the end of the first week, and at this stage the main nitrogenous component of urine was urea. However, with increasing ketosis the excretion of urea decreased, and by the end of the third week the majority of urine nitrogen was appearing as ammonia and this continued until the ketosis was relieved by giving glucose. This was done covertly at day 50 to see if the patient experienced any change in hunger, but none was noted. When the glucose was increased to 45 g daily she was nauseated, but at this stage it became necessary to increase her potassium supplement, which may have contributed to the nausea.

This study shows several features relevant to protein sparing in the fasting patient. The most important is to observe how, in the course of the starvation period, nitrogen is progressively more efficiently conserved until after about 5 weeks it is only 2.5 g/day on average, and most of this is ammonia. At this stage a trivial amount of glucose, providing only 60 kcal, causes the ammonia excretion to fall from about 1.8 g to 0.9 g ammonia nitrogen/day, and this appears as a "protein-sparing" effect. Addition of a further 30 g of glucose abolishes the ketosis in the last 10 days of the study, with a further improvement in nitrogen balance. Thus under conditions of severe energy and protein loss it is easy to show a protein-sparing effect of small amounts of glucose, as Jeejeebhoy (1976) shows in patients on parenteral nutrition. Had this amount of glucose been given at the beginning of the study it is very unlikely that any effect on nitrogen balance would have been evident, and we do not know if the protein sparing effect would have been different had protein, rather than glucose, been given.

Fig. 7.4 also illustrates the fluctuations in nitrogen excretion which occur even when the patient is maintained on a completely rigid protocol. Nitrogen retention over short periods does not provide evidence of protein synthesis, especially when the level of nitrogen input is suddenly increased, since under these conditions the urea pool may expand. It must be emphasised again that nitrogen balance studies are notoriously demanding: even if input is parenteral it is

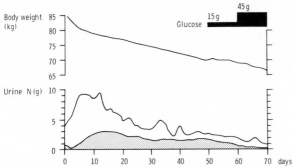

Fig. 7.4. Body weight and urine nitrogen losses in a patient on total starvation (only water, mineral and vitamin supplements) for 7 weeks. At day 50 she was given 15 g glucose daily, and at day 60 this was increased to 45 g daily. Stippled area shows the portion of urine nitrogen as ammonia (Halliday et al., unpublished).

necessary to check how much of the fluid which started in the infusion bottle finished in the patient (Millard, 1977), since small errors in estimating intake or output produce large errors in the calculated balance.

7.2.3. Conventional reducing diets

The conventional dietary management of obesity is to advise the patient to eat normal food, but to reduce the quantities of certain foods, especially those of high energy density. The objective is to reduce energy intake below the normal level of energy expenditure, so the deficit is made up by burning the energy stores of the body, chiefly fat.

The advantages of this system are that it is relatively safe and inexpensive: since normal food is taken it is unlikely that any significant dietary deficiencies will occur except the intended deficiency of energy, and the argument in favour of eliminating items like sugar from the diet is that the resulting deficit will be purely of energy and not of any other nutrient. If carbohydrate foods generally are restricted it is likely that fat normally taken with carbohydrate (butter with bread, frying oil with potato chips) will also be reduced (Yudkin, 1974), but the effectiveness of low carbohydrate diets depends on total energy intake being reduced: you can "eat fat and grow slim" (Mackarness, 1958) only if in the process you eat fewer calories. Advice and recipes for such diets are readily available (Craddock, 1973) and doctors probably underestimate their effectiveness. Most patients who consult a doctor about losing weight have already tried such a diet from a magazine or slimming club, so doctors tend to see patients in whom this type of diet has failed.

If these conventional diets fail to produce the expected weight loss there are several possible explanations. Commonly the explanation is that the estimate of weight loss was impossibly optimistic (Ford et al., 1977). Slimming club leaders have a natural tendency to overstate the effectiveness of the diet they advocate and to draw attention to the more successful members of their groups, thus a newcomer to the group who "only" loses 2 lb (1 kg) in a week may go away disappointed, and despair when the following week it is an even smaller loss. This difficulty is fairly easily dealt with by rational explanation, and if the patient does not believe that a rate of loss between 1 and 2 lb/week is as much as can be expected in the long run experience will soon demonstrate that this is so.

If the problem is that the patient loses no weight at all over many weeks despite keeping to the diet this must mean that the anticipated energy deficit has not been generated, either because the patient has not observed the dietary restrictions sufficiently closely, or because a normal reducing diet meets the energy requirements of the patient. Reference to Fig. 5.8 will show that women may indeed have an average daily energy expenditure of 1200 kcal (5 MJ) daily, so the "normal" reducing diet for women of 1200 kcal (5 MJ) would not be expected to cause weight loss. The consequence of this range of energy expenditure on rate of weight loss is indicated in Fig. 7.5.

Most patients on a diet supplying 800 kcal/day will lose about 4—5 kg in 3 weeks, but some will lose more than 9 kg and some less than 2 kg. If immediately before coming into a metabolic ward for investigation of obesity the patient has an eating binge the weight loss tends to be greater (non-dieters in Fig. 7.5), but whether they have or have not been keeping to the diet before admission there is still a large scatter in weight loss, which corresponds very closely with the scatter in metabolic rate shown in Fig. 5.8. Therefore failure to lose weight on a diet supplying (say) 1200 kcal daily is not neces-

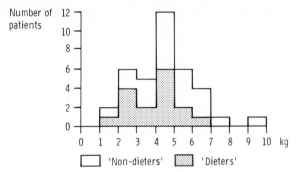

Fig. 7.5. Weight loss over 3 weeks in 37 women who were maintained on a diet supplying 800 kcal (3.4 MJ) daily. "Dieters" were those who had been keeping to this diet during the week before admission to hospital.

sarily evidence of "cheating", but this is often the explanation (Miller and Parsonage, 1975).

The desirable qualities in a reducing diet are therefore that it should create an energy deficiency (but not a deficiency of any essential nutrient) and that it should be well tolerated. Many attempts have been made to combine these characteristics, but it is probably impossible to devise any single diet which has either of these characteristics for all patients and still more impossible to find one which satisfies both criteria. No diet has yet been shown to increase metabolic rate out of proportion to its energy content, i.e. to have a specific thermogenic effect. High protein diets do not have this effect (Swift et al., 1957; Garrow and Hawes, 1972). Kasper et al. (1975) cite evidence that metabolism is increased by a high fat diet, but this view has yet to be confirmed. Reuben (1976) suggests that a high fibre diet inhibits the absorption of energy from the gut, but this effect is small and applies at least as much to other nutrients as to energy (Southgate and Durnin, 1970). Therefore the problem is to find a low energy diet which is acceptable. For the same total energy intake, small frequent meals are usually more acceptable than infrequent large meals (Durrant et al., 1978), but it is not clear if the frequency of meals actually affects the weight gained or lost on iso-energetic diets. Fabry et al. (1974) and Metzner et al. (1977) found that obese people reported taking fewer meals per day than lean people, and Fabry (1973) and Debry et al. (1973) found obese subjects lost weight more rapidly when a reducing diet was given in several meals than when it was given as few meals, but Finklestein and Fryer (1971), Young et al. (1971) and Durrant et al. (1978) did not confirm this. Differences in lipogenesis can be demonstrated in nibbling or gorging animals, but there is great variation in response between rats and mice (Palmquist et al., 1977). An interesting study is reported by Mahler (1972) who found that overfed students gained more weight when fed a carbohydrate supplement providing an extra 1800 kcal (7.5 MJ) as a single dose than when it was given in 16 equal doses at hourly intervals. In interpreting these studies it is necessary to consider that the students may have altered their pattern of food intake at other times, since the interpretation otherwise implies that a regimen of frequent meals causes a greater energy expenditure than one with few meals of the same total energy content, but no direct evidence of this phenomenon is available.

Kempner et al. (1975) report amazing success in treating 106 obese patients with what they term a "rice/reduction diet programme". This is a low energy, low sodium diet dispensed daily at "rice houses" to which the patients report. Urine sodium and chloride are measured, so defaulters are easily unmasked; their sin is revealed by posting of urinalysis results in the rice houses with high values circled in red! Obviously this programme requires a total dedication by the patients, but those dedicated enough to stay in the programme do well: the proportion of drop-outs, and the long-term results are not reported.

7.2.4. Psychotherapy in the treatment of obesity

A psychotherapist (or a general physician) who treats an obese patient may have one of two objectives: either it may be to modify the patients attitude to his obesity so that he is not distressed by it, or alternatively to modify his attitude to eating so that he is better able to adhere to a reducing diet. It is obvious that these objectives are to some extent conflicting, and the line which is appropriate depends on the disability which the obesity causes and the likelihood that this will be relieved by weight loss (see 7.1.4). Merely to provide psychotherapy to obese patients to relieve their psychological stresses, but without seeking to affect food intake, has no effect on their weight (Hall et al., 1977). A patient who is in the normal range of weight but desperately wishes to be thinner needs psychotherapy to deflect her (since it is usually a teenage girl) from this ambition. It is difficult to measure the success of this type of treatment, but since it is not treatment for obesity it will not be discussed further here.

Behavioural modification has been hailed as the great new advance in the treatment of obesity since the publication by Stuart (1967) of extremely good weight loss in 8 patients who received intensive treatment along these lines for one year. Stuart (1976) reviews the progress in this field, and nobody has been able to reproduce his excellent results in a large series. The lesson seems to be that different people respond to different regimens: just as there are those who will leave home and subject themselves to the tyranny of the rice house (Kempner et al., 1975) so there are patients willing to record in minute detail the circumstances in which they eat, and consequently eat less. Innumerable publications have appeared in the last few years in which the ways in which patients can bring pressure to bear on themselves or each other are described. Patients may agree that treats must be contingent upon keeping to prescribed eating behaviour (Paulsen et al., 1976), they may be paid for weight loss (Hall et al., 1977), and this tends to improve results at least while the contingency contracting arrangement is in force (Abrahamson, 1977). Support from members of a group is helpful to some (Blake, 1976), and even contact with a therapist by telephone (Lindstrom et al., 1976) seems to be as effective as personal contact. In patients who are very susceptible to food cues it is helpful if they can identify and avoid such stimuli (Paulsen et al., 1976). However, all this requires some degree of sophistication on the part of the patient, and behaviour therapy flourishes mostly in the middle classes (Weisenberg and Frey, 1974). It is hoped that a means of permanently rendering obese patients more amenable to dietary restriction will be found, but no sure method of achieving this objective has been published so far.

7.3. The drug treatment of obesity

In the United Kingdom the cost to the National Health Service of drugs promoted for the treatment of obesity was about £ 2.5m in 1973 and about £ 3.5m in 1975. In the survey reported by Ashwell (1973) 43% of women and 18% of men attending a doctor for treatment of obesity were prescribed some pill: usually this was intended as an anorectic.

7.3.1. Anorectic drugs

The pharmacology of anorectic drugs has been expertly reviewed by Garattini and Samanin (1976) and Silverstone (1975). Undoubtedly they decrease hunger, but their potency in this respect tends to decrease with time. Most published drug trials are of very short duration, or have such high drop-out rates that it is impossible to assess the effectiveness of anorectic drugs in producing long-term weight loss. The best published trial is probably that of Steel et al. (1973) who compared various combinations of fenfluramine, phentermine and placebo in groups of 35 patients for each treatment protocol. The trial lasted 36 weeks and is unique in a trial of such size and duration in that more than half the patients in each of the 5 treatment protocols completed the course. The work involved in a trial of this sort is very great. Generally anorectic drugs work best if used intermittently (Munro et al., 1968), but fenfluramine is unsuitable for intermittent use since depression may follow sudden cessation of this drug (Steel and Briggs, 1972).

A new anorectic drug is mazindol, which has been tested by various authors (Heber, 1975; Sanders and Breidahl, 1976; MacLay and Wallace, 1977; Walker et al., 1977), but it does not seem to be superior to the older anorectics such as phentermine or diethylpropion (Smith et al., 1975).

Typical results of trials of anorectic drugs against placebo are that by 20 weeks the patients on the active drug will on average lose 10 kg, while those on placebo lose 5 kg. An extra loss of 5 kg is not to be despised, but there is no information about the subsequent course of patients in whom the anorectic drug has lost its potency. My impression is that such patients do worse than those who never had anorectic drugs, but this is an important point on which we have no information. Patients who have had experience of dieting both with and without the assistance of an anorectic drug usually report that in the long term they find dieting without drugs is preferable (Ashwell, 1973). The best that an anorectic drug can do is to remove hunger, and it is clear that hunger is only one of many reasons for patients defaulting on reducing diets. Keeping to a reducing diet, without any drug treatment, also reduces hunger (Durrant et al., 1978).

7.3.2. Thermogenic drugs

It is logical to seek drugs which increase energy expenditure (thermogenic) as well as those which decrease hunger (anorectic). Many have been tried, but the one which is most easily controlled is tri-iodothyronine. The clinical use of this drug is reviewed by Garrow (1974b) and Bray (1976). In summary, it is ineffective in producing weight loss in non-toxic doses unless the diet is also strictly controlled. It is debatable if it is justifiable to use it in patients who have a low metabolic rate, although no thyroid abnormality can be shown. The use of high doses is associated with large losses of lean tissue, but a dose of about 120 μg daily is usually safe and sometimes useful.

7.3.3. Other drugs and placebos

Diuretics are commonly misused to produce weight loss in obese patients, sometimes because they complain of premenstrual swelling and tense breasts. It is ineffective (Preece et al., 1975) and deflects the patient's attention from the fundamental problems of energy balance.

Human chorionic gonadotrophin has its advocates (Asher and Harper, 1973) despite many controlled trials showing it to be ineffective (Stein et al., 1976; Young et al., 1976; Shetty and Kalkhoff, 1977).

7.4. Exercise in the treatment and prevention of obesity

Obese people usually eat no more than lean ones (Ries, 1973), increased body weight increases the energy cost of some activities (Mahadeva et al., 1953), so it is tempting to conclude that "heaviness is associated with diminished physical activity" (Thomson et al., 1961) and hence "an exercise programme is an important part of the management of the obese patient" (Allen and Quigley, 1977).

Those who review the effects of physical activity are rarely dispassionate. Some academics are opposed to exercise: they resented compulsory games at school at which they performed indifferently and which interfered with their scholastic activities, and they have never got over it. In the opposing camp are professional physical educators who promote exercise and fitness with an evangelical fervour which transcends scientific judgement. I am not committed to either extreme view: in so far as I achieved any distinction as an undergraduate it was at tennis, golf and squash, but I am not at all convinced by the claims made by Allen and Quigley (1977) about the usefulness of exercise in the treatment of obesity. I am impressed by the evidence that exercise protects against coronary thrombosis (Morris et al., 1977) and has other metabolic, social and psychological benefits, but this book is about energy balance and obesity, so I will concentrate on the effects of exercise in that context.

7.4.1. Effects on energy balance

The increase in energy expenditure which can be produced by physical activity was discussed in Section 5.2, and the relative effects of activity and other factors on energy output are summarised in Section 5.4. The energy expended in physical activity in that section of the population not engaged in major athletics (that is, the vast majority of people) is less than the range of variation of energy expenditure found within groups of the same age, weight and lifestyle. Thus it is unlikely that the difference observed between the high and low intake groups studied by Morris et al. (1977) could be accounted for by differences in exercise, since the difference in mean intakes of the groups is 1370 kcal (5.7 MJ)/day. However, the difference between the observed intake of men who developed coronary heart disease and the expected intake *for men of the same height* was only 177 kcal (0.74 MJ) daily, which might well be attributable to differences in physical activity.

This is not to say that a difference of 177 kcal/day is negligible in terms of energy balance: other things being equal it could be a highly important difference. The problem is that we have very little idea how equal other things are. It is very difficult to say what effect (if any) physical activity has on food intake. The study of Mayer et al. (1956) which claimed to show that food intake was *increased* when activity fell from "normal activity" to "sedentary activity" is unconvincing when studied in detail. An analysis of this work is given in Section 3.3. We do not even know if the main contribution of muscular activity is in "exercise"such as walking, running or swimming, or merely in maintaining muscle tone (DeVries et al., 1976).

The influence of physical exercise in the treatment of obesity is discussed in Section 5.2. The publications reviewed there will not be discussed again: the conclusion is that most proponents of exercise have calculated the *gross* cost of the imposed activity and neglected to subtract the energy cost of what the subjects would otherwise have been doing, and have thus been disappointed with the results. It is true that the increased metabolic rate induced by exercise does not immediately fall to basal when the exercise ceases, but the investigation of Courtice and Douglas (1935) shows that it requires a lot of hard work to produce a measurable effect a few hours later, and our own results by direct and indirect calorimetry tend to confirm this conclusion.

Almost everyone advises obese patients to take more exercise as well as reducing food intake and this is good advice, because exercise brings benefits other than weight reduction (Sullivan, 1976). The suggestion that weight can be effectively lost by exercise without dietary restriction is not supported by published results (Gwinup, 1975), at least in the majority of obese patients who are enrolled in such a trial. Lewis et al. (1975) describe 45 men, aged 47 ± 8.6 years, who habitually ran 38.8 ± 19.4 miles/week, which shows that this is possible, but it is certainly unusual. When Lewis et al. (1976) enrolled 22 obese women aged 44 ± 6.8 years in a weight reduction programme involving both diet and exercise they lost 4.2 kg in 17 weeks. Their food intake was not known, but it is possible to calculate that the increased energy expenditure attributable to the exercise programme accounted for about 19% of the energy deficit estimated from the change in body weight and composition: Zuti and Golding

(1976) compared the effect of diet, exercise, or both, on the weight loss of 25 women over a period of 16 weeks. Each protocol was designed to produce a daily energy deficit of 500 kcal (2 MJ). At the end of the study the weight loss was not significantly different in the 3 treatment groups and averaged 11 lb (5 kg). Estimates of body composition were reported to show that in the groups with exercise there was actually a gain in lean tissue and a loss of fat greater than that obtained by diet alone. The validity of this conclusion rests on the accuracy of the measurements of body composition. For reasons set out in Chapter 6 it is very difficult to make reliable estimates of change in body composition which will give a true picture of the composition of a loss of only 5 kg. Perhaps I am prejudiced by a previous publication by the same authors (Zuti and Golding, 1973) in which body fat was "predicted" by a formula involving wrist diameter multiplied by the factor 6.358583. I doubt if anyone can measure the diameter of a wrist with an accuracy (or precision, see Section 2.5) better than 1%, so I would have more confidence if this constant had been quoted as 6.4, or possibly 6.36.

Girandola (1976) found that 20 college women who exercised at fairly high intensity tended to gain weight, but at lower intensity for longer periods they tended to lose weight. This is consistent with our ideas on the effect of exercise on storage of muscle glycogen. The problem of high intensity exercise does not arise with very obese patients: it requires very careful gradation of exercise load to enable them to achieve any reasonable level of activity (Foss et al., 1976).

7.4.2. Exercise in preventing obesity

Despite the meagre evidence that physical activity can make a significant effect on energy expenditure, there is reason to believe that it may have a disproportionate effect in preventing obesity. This is because in addition to the small effect on energy output, a regular programme of activity has an effect on general lifestyle which is difficult to define or measure. However, it is not too fanciful to suppose that if long-term control of body weight is largely cognitive (see 6.5) then it is important to ensure that warning signals are received when weight increases. One should not rely on clothes which are easily replaced with a larger size. However, if someone takes a pride and pleasure in competence at some sport, the decreased physical fitness associated with obesity will be a noticeable handicap in most sports. An exception is dinghy sailing, in which with increasing age and affluence the size of boat tends to increase and the advantages of lightness decrease. It would be interesting to compare the lifetime weight curves of dinghy sailors and cross-country runners.

7.5. Surgical treatment for obesity

The massively obese patient is in a desperate situation, and it often happens that he and his physician give up hope of controlling the situation without recourse to surgery. This is not a decision to be taken lightly, because the patients who are sufficiently obese to be considered for surgery are sufficiently obese to be poor surgical risks. However, surgeons are not by nature diffident or timid, and vast numbers of operations for obesity have been performed and are described in the literature. A brief summary of the results is given below.

7.5.1. Jejunoileal bypass

By far the most commonly performed operation for obesity is some form of jejunoileal bypass. The majority of the small bowel is short-circuited, so the absorptive area between the stomach and colon is greatly reduced. The results of this operation were reviewed in a symposium issue of the *American Journal of Clinical Nutrition*, Vol. 30, 1977. The operation has its risks, but so has obesity, so the problem is to balance the two (Faloon, 1976). Weight loss is usually dramatic and sustained, and surgeons of great experience still believe that the explanation is that the food which the patients eat is less well absorbed after the operation (Woodward et al., 1975). It is true that food is less well absorbed, but this is only a minor cause of the weight loss. Mulcare et al. (1970) showed that the loss of energy in the faeces was not sufficient to explain the observed energy deficit, so the principal cause of weight loss must be a reduced food intake. This fact has been rediscovered by Pilkington et al. (1976) and Bray et al. (1976a). The malabsorption, apart from the beneficial effect of dissuading the patient from eating too much, also involves loss of minerals, particularly magnesium (Swenson et al., 1974; Lipner, 1977) and vitamins (Juhl et al., 1974). The best proportions of gut to leave in circuit is still a matter of debate between surgeons (Baddeley, 1977). The operation seems to increase the tendency to form gall stones (Neshat and Flye, 1975; Bruusgaard et al., 1976; Morin and Barry, 1976). Studies on the composition of the weight loss give conflicting answers, which is not surprising in view of the heterogeneity of the material and errors in the methods. Scott et al. (1975) conclude that the tissue lost is mostly fat, but Carlmark et al. (1975) publish results which show a greater reduction in lean tissue than fat. Generally the psychological state of the patients is improved after the operation (Brewer et al., 1974; Solow et al., 1974; Crisp et al., 1977).

The main disadvantage of this operation is that it leaves the patient with a significant degree of malabsorption, especially for fat, and consequently at risk to develop the problems associated with malnutrition: liver damage and vitamin and mineral deficiencies. In my view it is not an adequate answer for the surgeon to say that with careful follow-up and supervision of the diet these complications can be controlled, even though this statement may be true. With careful follow-up and supervision of the diet the operation would not have been necessary in the first place: it was because these patients were unable to follow dietary advice that the operation was performed.

7.5.2. Gastric bypass

If it is accepted that the action of the jejunoileal bypass is mainly to limit food intake and its disadvantages arise from the malabsorption of essential nutrients, it is logical to seek the benefits of the limited intake by means of a gastric bypass operation. This was pioneered by Mason and Ito (1969), but has only recently gained popularity. The principle is to reduce the capacity of the stomach by means of an operation similar to a gastrectomy, but bypassing rather than resecting the lower part of the stomach. The anastomosis is made between the small pouch in the fundus of the stomach and the jejunum, so virtually no absorptive area is lost, but the stomach capacity is greatly reduced. Apart from Mason, few surgeons have long experience of this procedure, but it has a favourable report from those who have tried it (Soper et al., 1975; Hermreck et al., 1976; Hornberger, 1976; Cohen et al., 1977; Printen and Mason, 1977) and when series with either jejunoileal or gastric bypass are compared it seems that the gastric bypass, although rather more difficult to perform, has as good results in terms of weight loss, but with fewer complications (Alden, 1977).

7.5.3. Jaw wiring

Since a major hazard of gross obesity is the risk of death with surgery or anaesthesia, it seems sensible to achieve weight loss before surgery if possible. The original idea of jaw wiring (Garrow, 1974a) was that if compulsive eaters could be prevented from eating in response to stress it was likely that their weight would decrease, and some alternative response to stress would be learned meanwhile. The first part proved correct, but not the second. We now have experience of this procedure over a period of 4 years (Fordyce et al., 1978) and find it is a safe and effective means of producing weight loss, but usually this weight is regained unless something else is done to stop it. Rogers et al. (1977) and Wood (1977) have published series treated with jaw wiring, but have no long-term follow-up, so it may be that their experience will confirm ours. Probably the best policy for surgical treatment (in those cases where it is justified at all) is to achieve weight loss by jaw wiring and maintain it by performing a gastric bypass while the patient is still relatively thin.

7.5.4. Panniculectomy

Obese patients may pay to have local deposits of fat excised, but in my opinion they get poor value for their money. The removal of 5 kg of adipose tissue involves making large skin flaps, with a lot of scar tissue formed as the wound heals. Both cosmetically and from the viewpoint of health I have yet to see a local excision of fat which caused any improvement at all.

Plastic surgery to remove skin flaps over the pubis and in the axilla after massive weight loss are not included in this criticism.

7.5.5. Stereotactic surgery

It is interesting that direct stimulation of the lateral hypothalamus in man can cause hunger (Quaade, 1974). However, there is no justification for attacking the hypothalamus of obese patients either by stereotactic surgery (Quaade, 1974) or by radiation (Nadal et al., 1954).

7.6. Investigation of "refractory obesity" without laboratory or dietetic facilities

The main thrust of this book so far may be summed up in 4 statements: (1) Severe obesity is a serious and quite common disease which must reflect an imbalance between energy intake and output. (2) It can be treated effectively provided the patient is reasonably cooperative and the nature of the imbalance is identified, but inappropriate treatment is either ineffective (e.g. low carbohydrate diet for patient with low output) or harmful (e.g. starvation for patient with high output, or jejunoileal bypass for patient with low output). (3) Changes in body weight are not simply related to changes in energy balance, so even the most sincere patient, interviewed by the most competent dietitian, may give misleading information about the effect of a given reducing diet on the energy stores of the body. (4) In a metabolic ward, equipped with good facilities for energy balance studies, it is possible to measure the variables mentioned above and predict the effect of any given line of treatment.

All this is not much comfort to clinicians who have to deal with severely obese patients who are highly motivated to lose weight, but who do not have access to the laboratory facilities to make the diagnosis. Centres with such facilities are few and could not cope with all the patients who might be referred for investigation. The following do-it-yourself scheme of investigation is suggested for clinicians who wish to make an accurate diagnosis and take the appropriate action on their severely obese patients, but whose facilities are limited to those found in a small cottage hospital. It is not ideal, since it relies on changes in body weight to measure energy balance and this is invalid, even under the rigid test conditions proposed, in patients with oedema or who are on (or have recently stopped) diuretics. Also the scheme will not work with patients who cannot tolerate a diet of milk only for 3 weeks, or in whom such a diet causes diarrhoea.

The essential for any measurement of energy balance is to have a totally reliable estimate of intake. This is difficult to achieve with mixed diets. At the Clinical Research Centre we have many patients referred from other centres because they maintained weight on low energy diets, but on a diet of exactly the same nominal energy content, accurately dispensed in our metabolic ward, the same patient may lose weight quite rapidly and continue to do so. The implication is that the previous hospital did not control the diet sufficiently accurately, or that the additions to this diet from well-meaning relatives, patients, or even nursing orderlies, made nonsense of the whole investigation. It is quite wrong to conclude that these patients deliberately "cheated": they cannot be expected to know the difference between low energy fruit squash and diabetic fruit squash, or to refuse gifts of fruit if the sister in charge of the ward raises no objections.

The requirements for a do-it-yourself obesity investigation unit are therefore similar to those required for nursing infectious patients, but the objective is dietetic isolation rather than microbial isolation. Nurses are trained to understand the latter. If the hospital has excellent dietetic facilities these should be used to design a diet supplying 800 kcal (3.4 MJ) daily, with a constant protein, carbohydrate and sodium content to suit the tastes of the patient. In the absence of expert dietetic help a diet of two (imperial) pints of milk (1200 ml) will serve very well. Water, tea and coffee are allowed ad libitum, and low energy fruit squash (16 kcal/l, *not* diabetic squash containing sorbitol). If the patient is on treatment for hypertension with beta-blockers these can be continued at the same dosage, but it is undesirable that patients should be on any form of diuretic or purgative, or have stopped taking these immediately before admission. Treatment for diabetes by insulin or oral agents can continue, and antidepressant therapy should continue unchanged. Hypnotics at night can be given as required. Theoretically high dose steroids might affect weight loss in this test, but I have no first-hand evidence on this point.

If energy intake is rigidly held to 800 kcal (3.4 MJ) daily, and every possible step is taken to avoid shifts in body water content, then change in weight becomes (under these special circumstances) a fairly reliable index of energy expenditure *over the second and third week of the test*. Not very much information about metabolic rate comes out of weight change in the first week, since the glycogen stores of the body are equilibrating to the new situation. Rapid loss in this phase probably (but not always) indicates a fairly high carbohydrate intake before admission.

The plan, which should be explained to the patient beforehand, is this. For 3 weeks he (or she) will be kept in isolation in the same way as a patient with an infectious disease. The diet will consist solely of two pints of milk and acaloric fluids ad libitum, and no other food of any kind. The purpose of this is to attain a constant condition of the various energy stores of the body so that weight loss will indicate fat loss, it is not intended as a therapeutic diet which the patient will be expected to observe for the remainder of his or her life. If the patient thinks the scheme is absurd and incompatible with civil liberty (which it is) it may help to explain that it is the one adopted at a large research unit in London which is maintained at vast expense to the taxpayer, where the plan involves not only these dietary restrictions but many other inconvenient tests also.

If the patient agrees to the scheme he or she should be admitted to the isolation unit, given the diet, and weighed accurately daily by a responsible nurse. It causes less friction if the patient does not know the result of these daily weighings until the end of the test period: there will be fluctuations due to irregularity of bowel opening and possibly menstrual fluctuations. If there is rapid weight loss initially there will be subsequent disappointment when the slower component of weight loss is reached.

The strictness of isolation required obviously depends on the patient to some extent, but (within reasonable limits) the stricter the better. If decisions about the future treatment of an obese patient are going to depend on the result of the test — like a decision to have a bowel bypass operation — the inconvenience of 3 weeks of solitary confinement is not too high a price to pay. In practice there should be no problem about visits from close relatives who should be asked not to bring (or to leave in custody outside the ward) any outdoor clothes or containers which might conceal food. This is especially important if the family believes that the patient is a secret eater, but in fact the patient is losing little weight. Families are often unwilling to believe that an obese relative is not a glutton, so it is in the patient's interest that the relatives also should realise that, despite close security and a diet of only two pints of milk daily, not much weight was lost. However, it is very important that the obese patient should be isolated from other patients on unrestricted diets, since the temptation to provide sweets as a gesture of goodwill seems insuperable. One of the main chores for the nursing staff in this exercise is to collect excreta, or, where it is necessary for the patient to share toilet facilities with other patients, to escort the patient to and from these facilities to ensure that they obtain no extra food.

To interpret the results of the investigation the weight loss should be compared with the histogram in Fig. 7.5 which shows the weight loss in 37 women who were in our metabolic ward under similar surveillance for 3 weeks. Anyone who loses less than 3 kg in 3 weeks is certainly in the low output group and not suitable for any of the surgical treatments described in Section 7.5. Loss of more than 6 kg in 3 weeks on this regimen indicates high output (and probably an eating binge before admission). Management depends on the reason for the high intake, which is often social or psychological, but, if these factors cannot be improved, this is the category of patients in whom the surgical procedures will have the greatest success, at least in the short term. The majority will fall in the 3—6-kg loss in 3 weeks, and here subsequent management depends on how well tolerated the milk diet was. Some patients find it much better than they feared, it is cheap and simple, and they have seen that it is effective, so they may wish to continue on the same regimen. This may be a good idea, but the diet is deficient in iron and vitamins, so it requires a supplement of 200 mg ferrous sulphate and one vitamin compound tablet (BPC) or the equivalent. Theoretically the remaining deficiencies are in vitamin B_{12} and folate. These will not become important unless the diet is continued for some months: if this duration is contemplated the appropriate vitamins should be given. The other common problem with a milk-only diet is constipation, which should *not* be treated with irritant purgatives, since the bowel has little to expel. An inert bulk purgative will help, but it must be free from absorbable carbohydrate: bran contributes significantly to the energy content of these milk-based diets.

It should be clearly understood that the rate of weight loss to be expected if the patient wishes to continue with the milk diet is that observed in the third week, not the first. If weight loss is fairly rapid (say 5—6 kg over the 3 weeks, with more than 1 kg in the last week) progress will probably be quite good on 3 pints of milk (1800 ml) daily. At least this crude plan of investigation will indicate what type of treatment is likely to be effective and, more important, should prevent disastrously bad treatment. It is surprisingly well tolerated by patients, who will put up with a lot to escape the depressing cycle of vague diagnoses, inconclusive investigations and ineffective advice on treatment.

7.7. Factors affecting long-term prognosis

There is ample evidence that many patients who embark on treatment for obesity never achieve a result which satisfies them or anyone else. The general pessimism engendered by this observation has been discussed in 7.1.4, and my own conclusion is that, given reasonable cooperation from the patient, the prognosis is no worse in obesity than in any of the common diseases. If a clinician was offered a choice of patients, each of whom was unable to earn his living at some job involving light activity, which disease would he offer to treat most effectively? Of the possible causes of disability obesity would rank near the top of the list as one of the more treatable. It would be below trauma and acute infectious disease, but these conditions do not form a large part of the workload of the general physician anyway. The conditions which bring patients into hospital: myocardial infarction, strokes, cancers, chronic respiratory failure, chronic renal or hepatic failure, and all the degenerative diseases: surely compared with these the outlook in obesity is relatively good. However, it is obviously important to try to distinguish what factors affect prognosis in obese patients, since this may give a clue to aetiology and guidance for treatment.

7.7.1. Age of onset, severity and adipose cellularity

Court (1976) offers a scheme of classification for obesity in children with 5 types: those with endocrine disorders have a good prognosis if properly diagnosed and treated, those with inappropriate eating habits do well if suitably motivated to alter their eating habits, those in whom the obesity is symptomatic of physical or emotional disorder "may show a good response" if the cause is treatable, the fourth group consists of rare disorders of metabolism which are not treatable, and the fifth group is children with a "high set point for fat stores": the management for this last group is to avoid a weight reduction diet, anorectic drugs are not indicated, and the prognosis is that they are unlikely to lose their obesity. It is on the basis of obscure pronouncements of this sort that the reputation of the oracle at Delphi was founded, and the tradition was carried on by mediaeval astrologers and soothsayers, but it is not appropriate to a modern medical journal.

Obesity is always due to a positive energy balance, even in children with the most obscure inborn errors of metabolism. It may be that the accompanying mental or physical defect caused by that error in metabolism is so severe that the obesity is not worth worrying about, but talk about a "high set point" which can be recognised in retrospect by the lack of response to a lack of treatment is not much of a contribution to the advance of medical knowledge. To make progress it is necessary to have a testable hypothesis with a plausible chain of reasoning.

A good hypothesis is offered by Hirsch (1975): ". . . the hypothesis that obesity may be accompanied by an excessive number of adipocytes, possibly brought about by excess feeding in infancy and childhood, and that the excessive number of adipocytes remains constant and in some way causes a drive for maintaining the obese state." To this we may add the suggestion of Björntorp et al. (1975) "that when the fat cell size in different regions of an individual is known, as well as the total fat cell number, the success of an energy-reduced dietary regimen might be approximately predicted both in terms of remaining total body fat and in regional fat depot decrease." These are "good" hypotheses in the scientific sense: they suggest a testable model, and it is then open to anyone to test it by whatever means they can command. One of the predictions arising from the hypotheses stated above is that in general fat children will tend to remain fat, and thin children will tend to remain thin. Many papers have been published which claim to offer support to this prediction, but some are so conceived that they tell us nothing. For example Rimm and Rimm (1976) asked 73,532 women members of TOPS "Were you considered fat as a child?" The more overweight the women, the more likely they were to say they had been fat as a child: those who were 100% overweight at the time of the survey (the highest weight group reported) reported that about half had been fat as children, and in the less overweight groups a lower proportion answered the question Yes. The authors conclude "the data suggest that the risk of a fat child developing severe obesity is substantially greater than for a non-fat child."

This is poor reasoning, as the following analogy should show. Suppose 100 people were persuaded to spend an hour operating machines which each second recorded the cumulative total of a series of totally random numbers, which might be positive or negative. At the end of the hour the average score on all the machines would be close to zero, since the total of a random series of positive and negative numbers is zero if the number of tries is infinite. If, after a cup of coffee, the 100 people returned to their machines and continued to play for another hour, starting from the score left at the coffee break, the average score at the end of 2 h would still be zero, for the reasons given above. However, a suspicious competitor might note that the player with the highest score after 2 h also had a high score at the coffee break, and a sophisticated analysis of all the results would reveal that there was a highly significant correlation between the score at coffee and the final score. An independent inquiry might be set up to decide if the high-score machines had some bias from the start, or if their experience in the first hour somehow programmed them towards a similar bias during the second hour! In fact neither explanation is correct: this is the result you would expect with a retrospective analysis of random machines behaving randomly. The correct analysis, if bias is suspected, is to take the high- and low-scoring machines at coffee time, and see if the *change* in score during the second hour averages zero for both sets of machines. If it does not, then bias should be suspected.

The observations of Rimm and Rimm (1976) on weight, or of Knittle et al. (1977) on the cellularity of "obesity-prone" children neither prove nor disprove anything about prognosis, since they are retrospective studies. Well-designed prospective studies are very difficult to set up for human populations, but from the available evidence it is very difficult to predict what will happen to the weight of a fat baby. Poskitt and Cole (1977) reviewed a series of children who had been the subjects of a survey 4—5 years previously. Among the 5 obese toddlers 3 had been obese infants, but of the 9 obese infants only one was obese at 5 years. Mellbin and Vuille (1976) were unable to predict, from data on a large series of Swedish children, what characteristics of weight gain in infancy would identify those who would be obese at age 10.5 years. Ravelli et al. (1976) found that infants affected by the famine in North Holland during the last trimester of pregnancy or first months of life were less obese than average ($P <$ 0.005) but those whose mothers were exposed to famine in the first half of pregnancy were subsequently more likely to be obese ($P <$ 0.0005).

Charney et al. (1976) report that "infant weight correlates strongly with adult weight independently of other factors considered". In their series of 366 adults there were 32 whom they classified as obese. Of these 17 had been above the 90th percentile of weight for height as babies, 6 had been between the 25th and 75th percentile, and 9 had been below the 10th percentile. Sohar et al. (1973) are also impressed with the relative constancy of body weight in children. Among the 404 children aged 13—14 years whom they studied there were 39 who were 131—150% of ideal weight (their most obese category). Of these 17 had also been in this most obese category at age 6—7, but 6 had been in the 111—130% group, 12 had been in the 91—110% group, and 4 had been between 71 and 90% of ideal weight at age 6—7 years.

Wilkinson et al. (1977) reviewed 8000 children and selected those who were over the 97th percentile of weight-for-height at age 10 years. About half of these had not been overweight at age 5 years, and they were unable to find any characteristic of the weight curve of these children which would have predicted that they would be overweight at the age of 10 years. Whitelaw (1977) found a rather weak relationship between the skinfold thickness of babies at birth and at one year of age.

All this seems to show that while there are certainly fat babies who remain fat, there are also fat babies who become thin, and probably the majority of fat adults were not fat babies. Thus the adipose cell hypothesis may be true, but it cannot be the major determinant of subsequent obesity. Direct tests of the relationship between adipose tissue cellularity and subsequent obesity are hampered by difficulties in estimating the number of fat cells (see 6.2.3) and deciding if there is a pool of potential fat cells not detected by routine techniques (Ashwell, 1978b). The number of countable fat cells is not decreased in men who were undernourished early in life (Berglund, 1974) and when people of equal fatness are compared the number of countable fat cells is not related to the age of onset of obesity (Ashwell et al., 1975; Hirsch and Batchelor, 1977). Our own studies, either from the reported weight loss of women in relation to age of onset of obesity (Ashwell, 1975) or observed weight loss in relation to observed cellularity (Ashwell et al., 1975b) do not confirm the idea that early onset obesity or hyperplastic obesity is in general more difficult to treat. Johnson et al. (1976) found a slightly (but insignificantly) *greater* weight loss among obese patients with onset before the age of 12 years, compared with those of later onset.

7.7.2. Expectation, motivation and self-fulfilling prophecy

It is a tenable hypothesis that the most important prognostic factor in the treatment of obesity is a reasonable degree of optimism by both the doctor and the patient. Not an unreasonable amount: it is as disastrous to extrapolate the loss of 2 kg in the first week of dieting to a prediction of 40 kg loss in 20 weeks, as it is to prophesy total failure before treatment has even been tried. It is not surprising that doctors who believe that obesity is untreatable to any useful extent can produce statistics to confirm this attitude, but I have yet to read any documented report of an untreatable case of obesity. If the screening test proposed in 7.6 is applied a reasonable estimate will be obtained of the rate of weight loss which can be expected on a given diet. There are certainly circumstances in which obesity is not worth treating, either because it is too trivial, or because the patient has other disabilities such that the loss of excess weight would confer little net benefit. Pavel et al. (1969), in a very large series of cases in Bucharest, noted that weight loss was better than average in patients with heart failure or back pain. It is not necessary to invent complex metabolic explanations for this observation: overweight patients with heart failure or back pain have the disadvantages of obesity, and the advantages of weight loss, more clearly demonstrated to them than those who are less disabled. It is no therapeutic triumph to wait until factors such as these motivate patients. By providing realistic expectation and motivation, the doctor can afford to adopt a more optimistic outlook, and I believe that prophecy along these lines also tends to be self-fulfilling.

7.8. The fat liberation movement and the slimming industry

Many millions of pounds (and dollars) are spent annually persuading fashionable women to be slim, and popular diet books (but not this one) sell millions of copies. In reaction to this there is a National Association to Aid Fat Americans dedicated to removing the stigma of obesity in their society. Doctors may be caught in the crossfire between these two powerful pressure groups.

Concerning the social stigma of obesity there is no difficulty in my mind about the correct policy for the medical profession to adopt. Gross obesity is a handicap, but it is not a matter for moralising or ridicule. It was once fashionable to regard hunchbacks as figures of fun, and Punch in the traditional marionnette show of Punch and Judy is represented with a severe kyphosis which has now become so stylised that it is hardly recognisable, because hunchbacks are no longer considered funny. We have now advanced to the point where severe mental defect is no longer a suitable subject for comedy, and with luck in a few more years this enlightened view will extend also to the very obese. However, it is possible to show a normal degree of courtesy to obese patients without pretending that obesity is unimportant from the viewpoint of health. Young fat girls often come for treatment because they mind about the effect of their obesity on their social standing and self-esteem, not the long-term effects on their weight-bearing joints and surgical risks. In such circumstances it is possible to form an alliance with common objectives (namely a reasonable rate of weight loss) but from quite different motives. I see nothing disreputable in this expedient provided that it is understood that the doctor's concern is not based solely on considerations of social acceptability, and provided that nothing is done to damage still further the patient's self-esteem.

The opposite conflict arises when patients strive for an unphysiologically low weight in the service of fashion. Here again, it seems reasonable to use the range of weights (shown in Fig. 7.1) which are associated with longevity and general fitness. It is a great advantage to omit any mention of frame size, or time will be wasted in fruitless dispute about the frame size of a given patient. Anyone near the lower limit of that range can hardly expect medical help to go even lower.

7.9. The prevention of obesity

It is a platitude that since obesity is so difficult to treat it should be prevented. If the causes were better understood, or if some critical period in which susceptibility was determined was identified, then such advice might be applied. However, all attempts to predict obesity have a very high failure rate, so if preventive measures are adopted it is not clear to which special group they should be applied, and if they are to be assessed for effectiveness it is difficult to select a control group with which they can be compared.

Obesity runs in families, but as Garn and Clark (1976) point out, with correlations around 0.4 it is easy to be mislead into detecting "pseudo-hereditary" factors. Obesity in the *ob/ob* mouse is certainly genetically determined, yet transplanted fat cells from an obese mouse to a lean one become lean fat cells (Ashwell et al., 1977), so it seems to be the environment of the cells rather than their inherent genetic material which determines the expression even of genetic obesity. Certainly there are genetic factors which have a powerful

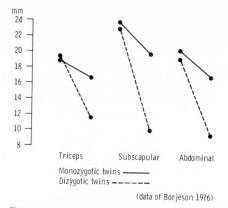

Fig. 7.6. Mean skinfold thickness at 3 sites in 40 pairs of monozygotic twins, and 61 pairs of dizygotic twins (data of Borjeson, 1976).

influence on the distribution of body fat (Garn, 1955): monozygotic twins have less difference in skinfold thickness between the two twins than if they are dizygotic (Borjeson, 1976). These striking results are shown in Fig. 7.6.

If it is true that we cannot identify particular individuals or particular stages of development, which require special attention to prevent obesity, the alternative is constant vigilance within reasonable limits. One stage at which moderately obese people are susceptible to dietary advice is during pregnancy, but the question of the management of obesity during pregnancy is highly emotive. The energy requirements of such women are well documented (Blackburn and Calloway, 1976), but some obstetricians take as their model the pregnant sow and advise diets designed on a truly heroic scale (Brewer, 1967). Any suggestion that obese women should gain less than 12 kg during pregnancy is regarded with great caution by most obstetricians, since in normal weight mothers small weight gain during pregnancy is associated with small-for-dates babies. However, the general rule does not apply to overweight mothers: they tend to gain less weight than average but produce bigger babies (Peckham and Christianson, 1971). Ketosis is bad for fetal growth, but it is both possible and ethical to maintain an overweight mother at constant weight during pregnancy without danger to the fetus. The energy cost of pregnancy is about 200 kcal (0.8 MJ)/day above non-pregnant requirements, so if the obese mother draws this modest contribution from her adipose tissue, instead of eating enough to maintain her adipose stores as well as her pregnancy, it will be to her advantage when the pregnancy is over.

7.10. Summary and conclusions

It is not possible to give a precise estimate of the prevalence of obesity without an agreed criterion for diagnosis, but about 20–30% of the adult population of Britain is above the "desirable" range of weight for height, and the prevalence of obesity is probably increasing. In such people weight loss would decrease the risk of diabetes, hypertension, gall bladder disease and (in certain groups) ischaemic heart disease and degenerative disease of weight-bearing joints. Obesity certainly increases the risks in surgery and childbirth. The younger and more severely overweight patients are most important to treat.

Most people who wish to lose weight do not at first seek medical advice: they try dieting on their own or with some slimming group. It is therefore useless for a doctor to expect that general dietary exhortation from him will succeed in a patient who has already tried this and failed. The prescription of anorectic drugs is not an adequate substitute for a proper assessment of the situation in a given patient.

The necessary steps for this assessment are set out in this book: to determine the likely benefit to the patient of weight loss, the reasons why previous attempts have failed, and a realistic estimate of the line of treatment which is likely to be effective and the rate of weight loss which this will achieve. If the patient can be convinced that this assessment is accurate, and that the effort is worthwhile, then a reasonable degree of optimism on both sides is both justified and necessary. However, if failure is prophesied at the outset, it will come to pass.

In my opinion surgical treatment of obesity is never justified until at least a rudimentary study of energy balance in the patient has been carried out. Any doctor with facilities for performing the surgery must have facilities for this investigation. Some patients being treated surgically did not need it, and some predictably will not benefit from it.

Although little progress has been made in the prevention of obesity, techniques for the study of energy balance have advanced very rapidly in the last few years, and with these technical advances has come a better understanding of the factors which predispose to obesity. The convergence of many disciplines on this problem has been most profitable. There is clearly no single cause for the positive energy balance which causes obesity, nor is there any single genetic or environmental factor which renders an individual immune to obesity, or which makes obesity inevitable.

In his play, "The Doctor's Dilemma", George Bernard Shaw paints an unflattering picture of the hypocricy and avarice of the medical profession: one of his characters attributes his commercial success to the slogan he adopts for all patients — "Cure Guaranteed." Such a claim is fraudulent for most of the conditions which a doctor has to treat, but with patience, an understanding of the principles of energy balance, a realistic but sympathetic attitude, and a fair degree of cooperation from the patient, such a claim can honestly be made for the great majority of cases of obesity.

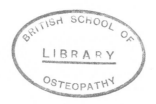

References

Abramson, E.E., 1977, Behavioural approaches to weight control: an updated review. *Behav. Res. Ther., 15*, 355–364.

Adam, J.M., Best, T.W. and Edholm, O.G., 1961, Weight changes in young men. *J. Physiol. (Lond.), 156*, 38P.

Adolph, E.F., 1947, Urges to eat and drink in rats. *Amer. J. Physiol., 151*, 110–125.

Alden, J.F., 1977, Gastric and jejunoileal bypass: a comparison in the treatment of morbid obesity. *Arch. Surg., 112*, 799–806.

Alexander, M.K., 1964, The postmortem estimation of total body fat, muscle and bone. *Clin. Sci., 26*, 193–202.

Allen, D.W. and Quigley, B.M., 1977, The role of physical activity in the control of obesity. *Med. J. Aust., 2*, 434–438.

Allen, T.H., Krzywicki, H.J. and Roberts, J.E., 1959, Density, fat, water and solids in freshly isolated tissues. *J. appl. Physiol., 14*, 1005–1008.

Alpers, D.H., 1977, Gastric bypass for obesity. *Gastroenterology, 72*, 976–977.

Anand, B.K., 1974, Neurological mechanisms regulating appetite. In: W.L. Burland (Ed.), *Obesity*, Churchill-Livingstone, Edinburgh, pp. 116–145.

Antonetti, V.W., 1973, The equations governing weight change in human beings. *Amer. J. clin. Nutr., 26*, 64–71.

Apfelbaum, M., 1976, The effects of very restrictive high protein diets. *Clin. endocr. Metab., 5*, 417–430.

Apfelbaum, M., Bostsarron, J. and Lacatis, D., 1971, Effect of caloric restriction and excessive caloric intake on energy expenditure. *Amer. J. clin. Nutr., 24*, 1405–1409.

Apfelbaum, M., Brigant, L. and Joliff, M., 1977, Effects of severe diet restriction on the oxygen consumption of obese women during exercise. *Int. J. Obesity, 1*, 387–393.

Aschoff, J. and Pohl, H., 1970, Rhythmic variations in energy metabolism. *Fed. Proc., 29*, 1541–1552.

Asher, W.L. and Harper, H.W., 1973, Effect of human chorionic gonadotropins on weight loss, hunger and feeling of well being. *Amer. J. clin. Nutr., 26*, 211–218.

Ashwell, M.A., 1973, A survey investigating patients' views on doctors' treatment of obesity. *Practitioner, 211*, 653–658.

Ashwell, M.A., 1975, The relationship of age of onset of obesity to the success of its treatment in the adult. *Brit. J. Nutr., 34*, 201–204.

Ashwell, M.A., 1978a, Commercial weight-loss groups. In: G. Bray (Ed.), *Recent*

198

Advances in Obesity Research, Vol. II, Newman, London, in press.

Ashwell, M.A., 1978b, The fat cell pool hypothesis. *Int. J. Obesity, 2*, 69–72.

Ashwell, M.A. and Etchell, L., 1974, Attitude of the individual to his own body weight. *Brit. J. prev. soc. Med., 28*, 127–132.

Ashwell, M. and Garrow, J.S., 1973, Full and empty fat cells. *Lancet, ii*, 1021.

Ashwell, M. and Garrow, J.S., 1975, A survey of three slimming and weight control organisations in the U.K. *Nutrition (Lond.), 29*, 347–356.

Ashwell, M. and North, W.R.S., 1978, Obesity, smoking habits and social class in a working population in London, in press.

Ashwell, M.A., Priest, P. and Bondoux, M., 1975a, Adipose tissue cellularity in obese women. I. Relation to the age of onset of obesity. II. Relation to the behaviour of the fat site on weight gain and loss. In: A. Howard (Ed.), *Recent Advances in Obesity Research. I. Proc. 1st int. Congr. Obesity*, Newman, London.

Ashwell, M.A., Priest, P., Bondoux, M. and Garrow, J.S., 1975b, Resistance to slimming: adipose tissue cellularity studies. *Proc. Nutr. Soc., 34*, 85A.

Ashwell, M., Priest, P. and Sowter, C., 1975c, Importance of fixed sections in the study of adipose tissue cellularity. *Nature (Lond.), 256*, 724–725.

Ashwell, M., Priest, P., Bondoux, M., Sowter, C. and McPherson, C.K., 1976, Human fat cell sizing – a quick, simple method. *J. Lipid Res., 17*, 190–192.

Ashwell, M., Meade, C.J., Medawar, P. and Sowter, C., 1977, Adipose tissue: contributions of nature and nurture to the obesity of an obese mutant mouse *(ob/ob)*. *Proc. roy. Soc. B, 195*, 343–353.

Ashwell, M., Chinn, S., Stalley, S. and Garrow, J.S., 1978, Female fat distribution – a photographic and cellularity study. *Int. J. Obesity*, in press.

Ashworth, A., 1974, Ad lib. feeding during recovery from malnutrition. *Brit. J. Nutr., 31*, 109–112.

Ashworth, A. and Wolff, H.S., 1969, A simple method for measuring calorie expenditure during sleep. *Pflügers Arch. ges. Physiol., 306*, 191–194.

Ashworth, N., Creedy, S., Hunt, J.N., Mahon, S. and Newland, P., 1962, Effect of nightly food supplements on food intake in man. *Lancet, ii*, 685–687.

Astwood, E.B., 1962, The heritage of corpulence. *Endocrinology, 71*, 337–341.

Atwater, W.O. and Benedict, F.G., 1899, Experiments on the metabolism of matter and energy in the human body. *Bull. U.S. Dept. Agric., 69*, 112 pp.

Atwater, W.O. and Benedict, F.G., 1905, *A Respiration Calorimeter with Applicances for the Direct Determination of Oxygen*, Carnegie Institution of Washington, Washington, D.C., Publication 42, 193 pp.

Baddeley, R.M., 1977, Modified jejunoileal bypass for obesity. *Brit. med. J., 2*, 1290.

Bae, J., Ting, E.Y. and Gioffrida, J.G., 1976, The effects of changes in body position of obese patients on pulmonary volume and ventilatory function. *Bull. N.Y. Acad. Med., 52*, 830–837.

Baird, I.McL., Parsons, R.L. and Howard, A.N., 1974a, Clinical and metabolic studies of chemically defined diets in the management of obesity. *Metabolism, 23*, 645–657.

Baird, I.McL., Silverstone, J.T., Grimshaw, J.J. and Ashwell, M.A., 1974b, Prevalence of obesity in a London borough. *Practitioner, 212*, 706–714.

Baker, G.L., 1969, Human adipose tissue composition and age. *Amer. J. clin. Nutr., 22*, 829–835.

Baker, J.A., Humphrey, S.J.E. and Wolff, H.S., 1967, Socially acceptable monitoring instruments (SAMI). *J. Physiol. (Lond.), 188*, 4P–5P.

Ball, M.F., Canary, J.J. and Kyle, L.H., 1967, Comparative effect of caloric restriction and total starvation on body composition in obesity. *Ann. intern. Med., 67*, 60–67.

Beaudoin, R. and Mayer, J., 1953, Food intakes of obese and non-obese women. *J. Amer. diet. Ass., 29*, 29–33.

Beeston, J.W.U., 1965, Determinations of specific gravity of live sheep and its correlation with fat percentage. In: J. Brozek (Ed.), *Human Body Composition*, Pergamon Press, Oxford, pp. 49–55.

Behnke, A.R., Feen, B.G. and Welham, W.C., 1942, The specific gravity of healthy men: body weight and volume as an index of obesity. *J. Amer. med. Ass., 118*, 495–498.

Bender, A.E. and Bender, D.A., 1976, Maintenance of weight loss in obese subjects. *Brit. J. prev. soc. Med., 30*, 60–65.

Benedict, F.G., 1930, A helmet for use in clinical studies of gaseous metabolism. *New Engl. J. Med., 203*, 150–158.

Benedict, F.G. and Benedict, C.G., 1933, *Mental Effort in Relation to Gaseous Exchanges, Heart Rate, and the Mechanics of Respiration*, Carnegie Institution of Washington, Washington, D.C., Publication 446, 83 pp.

Benedict, F.G., Miles, W.R., Roth, P. and Smith, M., 1919, *Human Vitality and Efficiency under Prolonged Restricted Diet*, Carnegie Institution of Washington, Washington, D.C., Publication 280, 701 pp.

Benoit, F.L., Martin, R.L. and Watten, R.H., 1965, Changes in body composition during weight reduction in obesity: Balance studies comparing the effect of fasting and a ketogenic diet. *Ann. intern. Med., 63*, 604–612.

Benzinger, T.H., Huebscher, R.G., Minard, D. and Kitzinger, C., 1958, Human calorimetry by means of the gradient principle. *J. appl. Physiol., 12, Suppl. 1*, 1–28.

Berg, K.H. and Isaksson, B., 1970, Body composition and nutrition of school children with cerebral palsy. *Acta paediat. (Uppsala), Suppl. 204*, 41–52.

Berglund, G., Björntorp, P., Sjöström, L. and Smith, U., 1974, Effects of early malnutrition in man on body composition and adipose tissue cellularity at adult age. *Acta med. scand., 195*, 213–216.

Beumont, P.J.V., George, G.C.W., Pimstone, B.L. and Vinik, A.I., 1976, Body weight and the pituitary response to hypothalamic releasing hormones in patients with anorexia nervosa. *J. clin. Endocr., 43*, 487–496.

Binnie, C.C., 1977, Obesity in general practice. Ten year follow-up of obesity. *J. roy. Coll. gen. Pract., 27*, 492–495.

Biron, P., Boyer, L., Brouillet, J., Boyer, A., Senecal, L. and Moisan, R., 1977, Dietary compliance in obesity: ketonuria versus weight loss. *Soc. occup. Med., 5*, 70.

Bistrian, B.R., Blackburn, G.L. and Scrimshaw, N.S., 1975, Effect of mild infectious illness on nitrogen balance in patients on a modified fast. *Amer. J. clin. Nutr., 28*, 1044–1051.

Bistrian, B.R., Winterer, J., Blackburn, G.L., Young, V. and Sherman, M., 1977a,

Effect of a protein-sparing diet and brief fast on nitrogen metabolism in mildly obese patients. *J. Lab. clin. Med., 89*, 1030–1035.

Bistrian, B.R., Blackburn, G.L. and Stanbury, J.B., 1977b, Protein sparing modified fast in the management of Prader–Willi obesity. *New Engl. J. Med., 296*, 774–779.

Björntorp, P., Carlgren, G., Isaksson, B., Krotkiewski, M., Larsson, B. and Sjöström, L., 1975, Effect of an energy-reduced dietary regimen in relation to adipose tissue cellularity in obese women. *Amer. J. clin. Nutr., 28*, 445–452.

Bjurulf, P., 1959, Atherosclerosis and body build with special reference to size and number of subcutaneous fat cells. *Acta med. scand., 166, Suppl. 349*, 29.

Blackburn, G.L., Bistrian, R. and Flatt, J.P., 1975, Role of a protein sparing fast in a comprehensive weight reduction programme. In: A. Howard (Ed.), *Recent Advances in Obesity Research, Vol. I*, Newman, London, pp. 279–281.

Blackburn, M.W. and Calloway, D.H., 1976, Energy expenditure and consumption of mature, pregnant and lactating women. *J. Amer. diet. Ass., 69*, 29–37.

Blair, B.F. and Haines, L.W., 1966, Mortality experience according to build at higher durations. *Trans. Actuarial Soc. Amer., 18*, 35–41.

Blake, A., 1976, Group approach to weight control: behaviour modification, nutrition and health education. *J. Amer. diet. Ass., 69*, 645–649.

Blaxter, K.L., 1971, Methods of measuring the energy metabolism of animals and interpretation of results obtained. *Fed. Proc., 30*, 1436–1443.

Blaxter, K.L., 1976, Energy utilization and obesity. In: G. Bray (Ed.), *Obesity in Perspective*, Fogarty International Center, U.S. Government Printing Office, Washington, D.C., pp. 127–135.

Blaxter, K.L., Brockway, J.M. and Boyne, A.W., 1972, A new method for estimating the heat production of animals. *Quart. J. exp. Physiol., 57*, 60–72.

Blitzer, P., 1976, Association between teen-age obesity and cancer in 56,111 women: all cancers and endometrial carcinoma. *Prev. Med., 5*, 20–31.

Bloom, P.B., Ross, D.L.F., Stunkard, A.J., Fox, S. and Stellar, E., 1970, Gastric and duodenal motility, food intake and hunger measured in man during a 24 hour period. *Amer. J. dig. Dis., 15*, 719–725.

Bloom, W.L., 1959, Fasting as an introduction to the treatment of obesity. *Metabolism, 8*, 214–220.

Bloom, W.L. and Eidex, M.F., 1967a, Inactivity as a major factor in adult obesity. *Metabolism, 16*, 679–684.

Bloom, W.L. and Eidex, M.F., 1967b, The comparison of energy expenditure in the obese and lean. *Metabolism, 16*, 685–692.

Boddy, K., Hume, R., White, C., Pack, A., King, P.C., Weyers, E., Rowan, T. and Mills, E., 1976, The relation between potassium in body fluids and total body potassium in healthy and diabetic subjects. *Clin. Sci., 50*, 455–461.

Bolinger, R.E., Lukert, B.P., Brown, R.W., Guevera, L. and Steinberg, R., 1966, Metabolic balance of obese patients during fasting. *Arch. intern. Med., 118*, 3–8.

Booth, D.A., 1976, Approaches to feeding control. In: T. Silverstone (Ed.), *Appetite and Food Intake*, Dahlem Konferenzen, Berlin, pp. 417–478.

Booth, D.A., 1977, Satiety and appetite are conditioned reactions. *Psychosom. Med., 39*, 76–81.

Booth, D.A. and Jarman, S.F., 1976, Inhibition of food intake in the rat following complete absorption of glucose delivered into the stomach, intestine or liver. *J. Physiol. (Lond.), 259*, 501–522.

Booth, D.A., Lee, M. and McAleavey, C., 1976, Acquired sensory control of satiation in man. *Brit. J. Psychol., 67*, 137–147.

Booth, R.A.D., Goddard, B.A. and Paton, A., 1966, Measurement of fat thickness in man: a comparison of ultrasound, Harpenden calipers and electrical conductivity. *Brit. J. Nutr., 20*, 719–725.

Boothby, W.M. and Berkson, J., 1933, In: G.A. Bray (Ed.), *Obesity in Perspective*, D.H.E.W., Washington, D.C., Appendix 4, Table 7.

Boothby, W.M. and Sandiford, I., 1929, Normal values for standard metabolism. *Amer. J. Physiol., 90*, 290–291.

Boothby, W.M., Berkson, J. and Dunn, H.L., 1936, Studies of the energy metabolism of normal individuals: a standard for basal metabolism with a nomogram for clinical application. *Amer. J. Physiol., 116*, 468–484.

Booyens, J. and Hervey, G.R., 1960, The pulse rate as a means of measuring metabolic rate. *Canad. J. Biochem., 38*, 1301–1309.

Borjeson, M., 1976, The aetiology of obesity in children. *Acta paediat. (Uppsala), 65*, 279–287.

Bradfield, R.B., 1971, A technique for determination of usual daily energy expenditure in the field. *Amer. J. clin. Nutr., 24*, 1148–1154.

Bradfield, R.B. and Jourdan, M.H., 1973, Relative importance of specific dynamic action in weight reduction diets. *Lancet, ii*, 640–643.

Bray, G.A., 1969a, Effect of caloric restriction on energy expenditure in obese patients. *Lancet, ii*, 397–398.

Bray, G.A., 1969b, Calorigenic effect of human growth hormone in obesity. *J. clin. Endocr., 29*, 119–122.

Bray, G.A., 1970a, Measurement of subcutaneous fat cells from obese patients. *Ann. intern. Med., 73*, 565–569.

Bray, G.A., 1970b, The myth of diet in the management of obesity. *Amer. J. clin. Nutr., 23*, 1141–1148.

Bray, G.A., 1974, Endocrine factors in the control of food intake. *Fed. Proc., 33*, 1140–1145.

Bray, G.A., 1976, *The Obese Patient*, Saunders, Philadelphia, Pa., 450 pp.

Bray, G.A. and Gallagher, T.F., 1975, Manifestation of hypothalamine obesity in man. *Medicine (Baltimore), 54*, 301–330.

Bray, G.A., Schwartz, M., Rozin, R. and Lister, J., 1970, Relationship between oxygen consumption and body composition of obese patients. *Metabolism, 19*, 418–429.

Bray, G.A., Barry, R.E., Benfield, J.R., Castelnuovo-Tedesco, P. and Rodin, J., 1976a, Intestinal bypass surgery for obesity decreases food intake and taste preferences. *Amer. J. clin. Nutr., 29*, 779–783.

Bray, G.A., Dahms, W.T., Greenway, F.L., Marriott, M., Molitch, M. and Atkinson, R., 1976b, Evaluation of the obese patient. *J. Amer. med. Ass., 235*, 2008–2010.

Bray, G.A., Fisher, D.A. and Chopra, I.J., 1976c, Relation of thyroid hormones to body weight. *Lancet, i*, 1206–1208.

202

Brewer, C., White, H. and Baddeley, M., 1974, Beneficial effects of jejunoileostomy on compulsive eating and associated psychiatric symptoms. *Brit. med. J., 4*, 314–316.

Brewer, T., 1967, Human pregnancy nutrition: a clinical view. *Obstet. and Gynec., 30*, 605–607.

Brobeck, J.R., 1948, Food intake as a mechanism of temperature regulation. *Yale J. Biol. Med., 20*, 545–552.

Brobeck, J.R., 1965, Exchange, control and regulation. In: W.S. Jamamoto and J.R. Brobeck (Eds.), *Physiological Controls and Regulation*, Saunders, Philadelphia, Pa., pp. 1–13.

Brown, G.A., Bennetto, H.P., Miller, D.S., Rigby, M., Stock, M.J. and Stirling, J.L., 1977, A D.I.Y. human calorimeter for £ 100. *Proc. Nutr. Soc., 36*, 13A.

Bruch, H., 1940, Obesity in childhood. III. Physiologic and psychologic aspects of the food intake of obese children. *Amer. J. Dis. Child., 59*, 739–781.

Bruusgaard, A., Sörensen, T.I.A., Justensen, T. and Kragg, E., 1976, Bile acid metabolism after jejunoileal bypass operation for obesity. *Scand. J. Gastroenterol., 11*, 833–839.

Bullen, B.A., Reed, R.B. and Mayer, J., 1964, Physical activity of obese and non-obese adolescent girls, appraised by motion picture sampling. *Amer. J. clin. Nutr., 14*, 211–223.

Bulow, J.M., Hansen, M. and Madsen, J., 1976, Variation in human subcutaneous adipose tissue blood flow. *Acta physiol. scand., 96*, 30A–31A.

Burch, P.R.J. and Spiers, F.W., 1953, Measurement of the γ radiation from the human body. *Nature (Lond.), 172*, 519–521.

Burke, B.S., 1947, The dietary history as a tool in research. *J. Amer. diet. Ass., 23*, 1041–1046.

Burkinshaw, L., Cotes, J.E., Jones, P.R.M. and Knibbs, A.V., 1971, Prediction of total body potassium from anthropometric measurements. *Hum. Biol., 43*, 344–355.

Buskirk, E.R., 1974, Obesity: a brief overview with emphasis on exercise. *Fed. Proc., 33*, 1948–1951.

Buskirk, E.R., Iampietro, P.F. and Welch, B.E., 1957, Variations in resting metabolism with changes in food, exercise and climate. *Metabolism, 6*, 144–153.

Buskirk, E.R., Thompson, R.H., Moore, R. and Whedon, G.D., 1960, Human energy expenditure studies in the National Institute of Arthritis and Metabolic Diseases Metabolic Chamber. 1. Interaction of cold environment and specific dynamic action. 2. Sleep. *Amer. J. clin. Nutr., 8*, 602–613.

Buskirk, E.R., Thompson, R.H. and Whedon, G.D., 1963a, Metabolic response to cold air in men and women in relation to total body fat content. *J. appl. Physiol., 18*, 603–612.

Buskirk, E.R., Thompson, R.H., Lutwak, L. and Whedon, G.D., 1963b, Energy balance in obese patients during weight reduction: influence of diet restriction and exercise. *Ann. N.Y. Acad. Sci., 110*, 918–940.

Cabanac, M. and Duclaux, R., 1970, Obesity: absence of satiety aversion to sucrose. *Science, 168*, 496–497.

Cabanac, M. and Rabe, E.F., 1976, Influence of a monotonous food on body weight regulation in humans. *Physiol. Behav., 17*, 675–678.

Cabanac, M., Duclaux, R. and Spector, N.H., 1971, Sensory feedback in regulation of body weight: Is there a ponderostat? *Nature (Lond.), 229,* 125–127.

Cahill, G.F., 1970, Starvation in man. *New Engl. J. Med., 282,* 668–675.

Cahill, G., 1978, Obesity and diabetes: the odd couple. In: G. Bray (Ed.), *Recent Advances in Obesity Research, Vol. II,* Newman, London, in press.

Calloway, D.H. and Spector, H., 1954, Nitrogen balance as related to caloric and protein intake in active young men. *Amer. J. clin. Nutr., 2,* 405–411.

Campbell, R.G., Hashim, S.A. and Van Itallie, T.B., 1971, Nutritive density and food intake in man. *New Engl. J. Med., 285,* 1402–1407.

Carlmark, B., Kromhout, D. and Reizenstein, P., 1975, Total body potassium measurements in 230 patients. *Scand. J. clin. Lab. Invest., 35,* 617–623.

Chan, H. and Waterlow, J.C., 1966, The protein requirement of infants at the age of about 1 year. *Brit. J. Nutr., 20,* 775–782.

Charney, E., Goodman, H.C., McBride, M., Lyon, B. and Pratt, R., 1976, Childhood antecedents of adult obesity. *New Engl. J. Med., 295,* 6–9.

Chien, S., Peng, M.T., Chen, K.P., Huang, T.F., Chang, C. and Fang, H.S., 1975, Longitudinal studies on adipose tissue and its distribution in human subjects. *J. appl. Physiol., 39,* 825–830.

Chirico, A.M. and Stunkard, A.J., 1960, Physical activity and human obesity. *New Engl. J. Med., 263,* 935–940.

Cissik, J.H., Johnson, R.E. and Rokosch, D.K., 1972, Production of gaseous nitrogen in human steady state conditions. *J. appl. Physiol., 32,* 155–159.

Cohen, W.N., Mason, E.E. and Blommers, T.L., 1977, Gastric bypass for morbid obesity. *Radiology, 122,* 609–612.

Cohn, S.H., Ellis, K.J. and Wallach, S., 1974, In vivo neutron activation analysis: clinical potential in body composition studies. *Amer. J. Med., 57,* 683–686.

Cohn, S.H., Vaswani, A., Zanzi, I., Aloia, J.F., Roginsky, M.S. and Ellis, K.J., 1976, Changes in body chemical composition with age measured by total-body neutron activation. *Metabolism, 25,* 85–95.

Comstock, G.W. and Stone, R.W., 1972, Changes in body weight and subcutaneous fat thickness related to smoking habits. *Arch. environm. Hlth, 24,* 271–276.

Court, J.M., 1976, Childhood obesity. *Med. J. Aust., 1,* Special Suppl., 5–6.

Courtice, F.G. and Douglas, C.G., 1935–6, The effects of prolonged muscular exercise on the metabolism. *Proc. roy. Soc. B, 119,* 381–439.

Cowgill, G.R., 1928, The energy factor in relation to food intake: experiments on the dog. *Amer. J. Physiol., 85,* 45–64.

Craddock, D., 1973, *Obesity and its Management,* 2nd ed., Churchill-Livingstone, London.

Craddock, D., 1977, The free diet: 150 cases personally followed-up after 10 to 18 years. *Int. J. Obesity, 1,* 127–134.

Crisp, A.H. and McGuiness, B., 1976, Jolly fat: relation between obesity and psychoneurosis in general population. *Brit. med. J., 1,* 7–9.

Crisp, A.H., Kalucy, R.S., Pilkington, T.R.E. and Gazet, J.-C., 1977, Some psychosocial consequences of ileojejunal bypass surgery. *Amer. J. clin. Nutr., 30,* 109–120.

204

Croxson, M.S. and Ibbertson, H.K., 1977, Low serum triiodothyronine (t_3) and hypothyroidism in anorexia nervosa. *J. clin. Endocr., 44*, 167–174.

Culebras, J.M., Fitzpatrick, G.F., Brennan, M.F., Boyden, C.M. and Moore, F.D., 1977, Total body water and exchangeable hydrogen. II. A review of comparative data from animals based on isotope dilution and desiccation, with a report of new data from the rat. *Amer. J. Physiol., 232*, R60–R65.

Curtis Prior, P.B., 1975, Prostaglandins and obesity. *Lancet, i*, 897–899.

Dalen, N., Hallberg, D. and Lamke, B., 1975, Bone mass in obese subjects. *Acta med. scand., 197*, 353–355.

Davidson, I.W.F., Salter, J.M. and Best, C.H., 1960, The effect of glucagon on the metabolic rate of rats. *Amer. J. clin. Nutr., 8*, 540–546.

Debry, G., Rohr, R., Azouaou, R., Vassilitch, I. and Mottaz, G., 1973, Ponderal losses in obese subjects submitted to restricted diets differing by nibbling and by lipid carbohydrate. In: M. Apfelbaum (Ed.), *Energy Balance in Man*, Masson, Paris, pp. 305–310.

De Garine, I., 1972, The sociocultural aspects of nutrition. *Ecol. Food Nutr., 1*, 143–163.

De Looy, A.E., 1974, *Socially Acceptable Methods for Measuring Energy Expenditure in Man*, Ph.D. Thesis, University of London.

De Looy, A. and James, S., 1972, Electrical resistance and skin reaction to eight electrode jellies. *Proc. Nutr. Soc., 31*, 92A.

DeVries, H.A., Burke, R.K., Hopper, R.T. and Sloan, J.H., 1976, Relationship of resting EMG level to total body metabolism with reference to the origin of "tissue noise". *Amer. J. phys. Med., 55*, 139–147.

De Wardener, H.E., 1967, *The Kidney*, Churchill, London, 115 pp.

DeWys, W.D., 1977, Anorexia in cancer patients. *Cancer Res., 37*, 2354–2358.

DHSS/MRC Study Group, 1976, *Research on Obesity* (Ed., W.P.T. James), H.M.S.O., London, 94 pp.

Dickerson, J.W.T. and Widdowson, E.M., 1960, Chemical changes in skeletal muscle during development. *Biochem. J., 74*, 247–257.

Diethelm, R., Garrow, J.S. and Stalley, S.F., 1977, An apparatus for measuring the density of obese patients. *J. Physiol. (Lond.), 267*, 14P–15P.

Dixon, A.S. and Henderson, D., 1973, Prescribing for osteoarthritis. *Prescribers' J., 13*, 41–49.

Dole, V.P., Schwartz, I.L., Thorn, N.A. and Silver, L., 1955, The caloric value of labile body tissue in obese subjects. *J. clin. Invest., 34*, 590–594.

Donald, D.W.A., 1973, Mortality rates among the overweight. In: R.F. Robertson (Ed.), *Anorexia and Obesity*, R.C.P., Edinburgh, pp. 63–70.

Douglas, C.G., 1911, A method for determining the total respiratory exchange in man. *J. Physiol. (Lond.), 42*, 17P–18P.

Drenick, E.J., 1976, Weight reduction by prolonged fasting. In: G. Bray (Ed.), *Obesity in Perspective*, Fogarty International Center, U.S. Government Printing House, Washington, D.C., pp. 341–360.

Drenick, E.J., Swenseid, M.E., Tuttle, S.G. and Blahd, W.H., 1964, Prolonged starvation as a treatment for obesity. *J. Amer. med. Ass., 187*, 100–105.

Dublin, L.I., 1953, Relation of obesity to longevity. *New Engl. J. Med., 248*, 971–974.

Dugdale, A.E. and Payne, P.R., 1977, Pattern of lean and fat deposition in adults. *Nature (Lond.), 266*, 349–351.

Duncan, G.G., Jenson, W.K., Fraser, R.I. and Cristofori, F.C., 1962, Correction and control of intractable obesity. *J. Amer. med. Ass., 181*, 309–312.

Duncan, G.G., Jenson, W.K., Cristofori, F.C. and Schloss, G.L., 1963, Intermittent fasting in the correction and control of obesity. *Amer. J. med. Sci., 245*, 515–520.

Durnin, J.V.G.A., 1959, The use of surface area and of body weight as standards of reference in studies on human energy expenditure. *Brit. J. Nutr., 13*, 68–71.

Durnin, J.V.G.A. and Norgan, N., 1969, Variations in total body metabolism during "overfeeding" in man. *J. Physiol. (Lond.), 202*, 106P.

Durnin, J.V.G.A. and Passmore, R., 1967, *Energy Work and Leisure*, Heinemann, London, 165 pp.

Durnin, J.V.G.A. and Rahaman, M.M., 1967, The assessment of the amount of fat in the human body from measurement of skinfold thickness. *Brit. J. Nutr., 21*, 681–689.

Durnin, J.V.G.A. and Womersley, J., 1974, Body fat assessed from body density and its estimation from skinfold thickness: measurement on 481 men and women from 16–72 years. *Brit. J. Nutr., 32*, 77–97.

Durnin, J.V.G.A., Armstrong, W.H. and Womersley, J., 1971, An experimental study on the variability of measurement of skinfold thickness by three observers on twenty-three young women and twenty-seven young men. *Proc. Nutr. Soc., 30*, 9A–10A.

Durrant, M. and Mann, S., 1977, Investigations into patient responses to feeding low- and high-energy foods. *Proc. Nutr. Soc., 36,* 113A.

Durrant, M., Toft, R., Mann, S. and Garrow, J.S., 1977, Investigations into the role of fluid in energy balance. *Proc. Nutr. Soc., 36,* 17A.

Durrant, M.L., Stalley, S.F., Warwick, P.M. and Garrow, J.S., 1978, The effect of meal frequency on body composition and hunger during weight reduction. *Proc. Nutr. Soc.,* in press.

Dyer, A.R., Stamler, J., Berkson, D.M. and Lindberg, H.A., 1975, Relationship of relative weight and body mass index to 14 year mortality in the Chicago Peoples Gas Company study. *J. chron. Dis., 28*, 109–123.

Edelman, I.S. and Ismail-Beigi, F., 1974, Thyroid thermogenesis and active sodium transport. *Recent Progr. Hormone Res., 30*, 235–257.

Edholm, O.G., 1973, Energy expenditure and food intake. In: M. Apfelbaum (Ed.), *Energy Balance in Man*, Masson, Paris, pp. 51–60.

Edholm, O.G., 1977, Energy balance in man. *J. hum. Nutr., 31,* 413–431.

Edholm, O.G., Fletcher, J.G., Widdowson, E.M. and McCance, R.A., 1955, The energy expenditure and food intake of individual men. *Brit. J. Nutr., 9*, 286–300.

Edholm, O.G., Adam, J.M. and Best, T.W., 1974, Day-to-day weight changes in young men. *Ann. hum. Biol., 1*, 3–12.

Edwards, D.A.W., 1950, Observations on the distribution of subcutaneous fat. *Clin. Sci., 9*, 259–270.

Edwards, R.H.T., 1971, Percutaneous needle biopsy of skeletal muscle in diagnosis and research. *Lancet, ii*, 593–595.

Efiong, E.I., 1975, Pregnancy in the overweight Nigerian. *Brit. J. Obstet. Gynaec., 82,* 903–906.

Ellis, K.J., Shukla, K.K., Cohn, S.H. and Pierson, R.N., 1974, A predictor of total body potassium on man based on height, weight, sex and age: applications to metabolic disorders. *J. Lab. clin. Med., 83,* 716–727.

Entenman, C., Goldwater, W.H., Ayres, N.S. and Behnke, A.R., Jr., 1958, Analysis of adipose tissue in relation to body weight loss in man. *J. appl. Physiol., 13,* 129–134.

Fabry, P., 1973, Food intake pattern and energy balance. In: M. Apfelbaum (Ed.), *Energy Balance in Man,* Masson, Paris, pp. 297–303.

Fabry, P., Fodor, J., Hejl, Z., Braun, T. and Zvolankova, K., 1964, The frequency of meals: its relation to overweight, hypercholesterolaemia and decreased glucose tolerance. *Lancet, ii,* 614–615.

Faloon, W.W., 1976, An evaluation of risks – bypass versus obesity. *New Engl. J. Med., 294,* 159–160.

Fanger, P.O., 1970, *Thermal Comfort,* McGraw-Hill, New York, 244 pp.

Faust, I.M., Johnson, P.R. and Hirsch, J., 1977, Surgical removal of adipose tissue alters feeding behaviour and the development of obesity in rats. *Science, 197,* 393–396.

Feigin, R.D., Beisel, W.R. and Wannemacher, R.W., 1971, Rhythmicity of plasma amino acids and relation to dietary intake. *Amer. J. clin. Nutr., 24,* 329–341.

Fennessy, P.A., Harrison, M.H. and Davison, C., 1975, Nitrogen exchange across the lungs in resting man. *Resp. Physiol., 24,* 303–312.

Finkelstein, B. and Fryer, B.A., 1971, Meal frequency and weight reduction in young women. *Amer. J. clin. Nutr., 24,* 465–468.

Fisher, A., Waterhouse, T.D. and Adams, A.P., 1975, Obesity: its relation to anaesthesia. *Anaesthesia, 30,* 633–647.

Flatt, J.P.and Blackburn, G.L., 1974, Metabolic fuel regulatory system: implications for protein-sparing therapies during caloric deprivation and disease. *Amer. J. clin. Nutr., 27,* 175–187.

Fletcher, J.G. and Wolff, H.S., 1954, A lightweight integrating motor pneumotachograph (i.m.p.) with constant low resistance. *J. Physiol. (Lond.), 123,* 67P–69P.

Fomon, S.J., Thomas, L.N., Filer, L.J., Zeigler, E.E. and Leonard, M.T., 1971, Food consumption and growth of normal infants fed milk-based formulas. *Acta paediat. (Uppsala), Suppl. 223,* 36 pp.

Forbes, G.B., 1974, Stature and lean body mass. *Amer. J. clin. Nutr., 27,* 595–602.

Forbes, G.B. and Lewis, A.M., 1956, Total sodium, potassium and chloride in adult man. *J. clin. Invest., 35,* 596–600.

Forbes, G.B. and Reina, J.C. (1970) Adult lean body mass declines with age: some longitudinal observations. *Metabolism, 19,* 653–663.

Forbes, J.M., 1977, Eventual plateaux of body weights of sheep and cattle predicted by simulation models not incorporating set points for body fat content. *Proc. Nutr. Soc., 36,* 81A.

Forbes, R.M., Cooper, A.R. and Mitchell, H.H., 1953, The composition of the adult human body as determined by chemical analysis. *J. biol. Chem., 203,* 359–366.

Forbes, R.M., Mitchell, H.H. and Cooper, A.R., 1956, Further studies on the gross composition and mineral elements of the adult human body. *J. biol. Chem., 223,* 969–975.

Ford, M.J., Scorgie, R.E. and Munro, J.F., 1977, Anticipated rate of weight loss during dieting. *Int. J. Obesity, 1,* 239–243.

Fordyce, G.L., Garrow, J.S., Kark, A.E. and Stalley, S.F., 1978, Jaw wiring and gastric bypass in the treatment of severe obesity, in press.

Foss, M.L., Lampman, R.M. and Schteingart, D., 1976, Physical training program for rehabilitating extremely obese patients. *Arch. phys. Med., 57,* 425–429.

Fox, F.W., 1973, The enigma of obesity. *Lancet, ii,* 1487–1488.

Garattini, S. and Samanin, R., 1976, Anorectic drugs and brain neurotransmitters. In: T. Silverstone (Ed.), *Appetite and Food Intake*, Dahlem Konferenzen, Berlin, pp. 83–108.

Garn, S.M., 1955, Relative fat patterning: an individual characteristic. *Hum. Biol., 27,* 75–89.

Garn, S.M., 1961, Radiographic analysis of body composition. In: J. Brozek and A. Henschel (Eds.), *Techniques for Measuring Body Composition*, Nat. Acad. Sci. – Nat. Res. Council, Washington, D.C., pp. 36–58.

Garn, S.M. and Clark, D.C., 1976, Trends in fatness and the origins of obesity. *Pediatrics, 57,* 443–456.

Garnett, E.S., Barnard, D.L., Ford, J., Goodbody, R.A. and Woodhouse, M.A., 1969, Gross fragmentation of cardiac myofibrils after therapeutic starvation for obesity. *Lancet, i,* 914–916.

Garrow, J.S., 1965a, Total body potassium in Kwashiorkor and Marasmus. *Lancet, ii,* 455.

Garrow, J.S., 1965b, The use and calibration of a small whole body counter for measurement of total body potassium in malnourished infants. *W. Indian med. J., 24,* 73–81.

Garrow, J.S., 1974a, Dental splinting in the treatment of hyperphagic obesity. *Proc. Nutr. Soc., 33,* 29A.

Garrow, J.S., 1974b, *Energy Balance and Obesity in Man*, North-Holland Publ., Amsterdam, 335 pp.

Garrow, J.S., 1976, Upbringing, appetite and adult obesity. In: A.W. Wilkinson (Ed.), *Early Nutrition and Later Development*, Pitman Medical Publ., London, pp. 219–228.

Garrow, J.S., 1978, Regulation of energy expenditure in man. In: G.A. Bray (Ed.), *Second International Congress on Obesity*, Newman, London, in press.

Garrow, J.S. and Hawes, S.F., 1972, The role of amino acid oxidation in causing 'specific dynamic action' in man. *Brit. J. Nutr., 27,* 211–219.

Garrow, J.S. and Stalley, S.F., 1975, Is there a set point for human body weight? *Proc. Nutr. Soc., 34,* 84A.

Garrow, J.S. and Stalley, S.F., 1977, Cognitive thresholds and human body weight. *Proc. Nutr. Soc., 36,* 18A.

Garrow, J.S. and Warwick, P.M., 1978, Diet and obesity. In: J. Yudkin (Ed.), *The Diet of Man: Needs and Wants,* Applied Science Publishers, Barking, pp. 127–144.

208

Garrow, J.S., Murgatroyd, P., Toft, R. and Warwick, P., 1977, A direct calorimeter for clinical use. *J. Physiol. (Lond.), 267,* 16P.

Garrow, J.S., Durrant, M.L., Mann, S., Stalley, S.F. and Warwick, P., 1978, Factors determining weight loss in obese patients in a metabolic ward. *Int. J. Obesity*, in press.

Garry, R.C., Passmore, R., Warnock, G.M. and Durnin, J.V.G.A., 1955, *Studies on Expenditure of Energy and Consumption of Food by Miners and Clerks, Fife, Scotland, 1952,* Medical Res. Council, Sp. Rep. Ser. 289, H.M.S.O., London, 70 pp.

Garvey, A.J., Bosse, R. and Seltzer, C.C., 1974, Smoking, weight change and age. *Arch. environm. Hlth, 28,* 327–332.

Gentil, V., Lader, M.H., Kantamaneni, B.D. and Curzon, G., 1977, *Clin. Sci. mol. Med., 53,* 227–232.

Genuth, S.M., Castro, J.H. and Vertes, V., 1974, Weight reduction in obesity by outpatient semistarvation. *J. Amer. med. Ass., 230,* 987–991.

Gibbs, J. and Smith, G.P., 1977, Cholecystokinin and satiety in rats and rhesus monkeys. *Amer. J. clin. Nutr., 30,* 758–761.

Girandola, R.N., 1976, Body composition changes in women: effects of high and low exercise intensity. *Arch. phys. Med., 57,* 297–299.

Glick, Z., Shvartz, E., Magazanik, A. and Modan, M., 1977, Absence of increased thermogenesis during short-term overfeeding in normal and overweight women. *Amer. J. clin. Nutr., 30,* 1026–1035.

Gold, R.M., 1973, Hypothalamic obesity: the myth of the ventromedial nucleus. *Science, 182,* 488–490.

Goldblatt, P.E., Moore, M.E. and Stunkard, A.J., 1965, Social factors in obesity. *J. Amer. med. Ass., 192,* 1039–1044.

Goldman, R.F. and Buskirk, E.R., 1961, Body volume measurement by underwater weighing: description of a method. In: J. Brozek and A. Henschel (Eds.), *Techniques for Measuring Body Composition,* Nat. Acad. Sci., Washington, D.C., pp. 78–89.

Goldman, R.F., Haisman, M.F., Bynum, G., Horton, E.S. and Sims, E.A.H., 1976, Experimental obesity in man. Metabolic rate in relation to dietary intake. In: G. Bray (Ed.), *Obesity in Perspective,* Fogarty International Center, U.S. Government Printing Office, Washington, D.C., pp. 165–186.

Goldrick, R.B., Havenstein, N. and Whyte, H.M., 1973, Effect of caloric restriction and fenfluramine on weight loss and personality profile of patients with longstanding obesity. *Aust. N.Z. J. Med., 3,* 131–141.

Goldsmith, R., Miller, D.S., Mumford, P. and Stock, M.J., 1966, The use of long term measurement of heart rate to assess energy expenditure. *J. Physiol. (Lond.), 189,* 35P–36P.

Goodner, C.J. and Ogilvie, J.T., 1974, Homeostasis of body weight in a diabetes clinic population. *Diabetes, 23,* 318–326.

Gordon, T. and Kannel, W.B., 1973, The effects of overweight on cardiovascular diseases. *Geriatrics, 28,* 80–88.

Göschke, H., Stahl, M. and Thölen, H., 1975, Nitrogen loss in normal and obese subjects during total fast. *Klin. Wschr., 53,* 605–610.

Gour, K.N. and Gupta, M.C., 1968, Social aspects of overweight and obesity. *J. Ass. Phycns India, 16,* 257–261.

Grande, F., 1968, Energy balance and body composition changes. A critical study of three recent publications. *Ann. intern. Med., 68,* 467–480.

Gray, H. and Kallenbach, D.C., 1939, Obesity treatment: results in 212 outpatients. *J. Amer. diet. Ass., 15,* 239–245.

Grimes, W.B. and Franzini, L.R., 1977, Skinfold measurement techniques for estimating percentage body fat. *J. behav. Ther. exp. Psychiat., 8,* 65–69.

Greenberg, I., Kuehnle, J., Mendelson, J.H. and Bernstein, J.G., 1976, Effects of marihuana use on body weight and calorie intake in humans. *Psychopharmacologia (Berl.), 49,* 79–84.

Greenfield, N.S. and Fellner, C.H., 1969, Resting level of physical activity in obese females (Guest Editorial). *Amer. J. clin. Nutr., 22,* 1418–1419.

Grossman, S.P., 1976, Neuroanatomy of food and water intake. In: D. Novin, W. Wyrwicka and G.A. Bray (Eds.), *Hunger, Basic Mechanisms and Clinical Implications,* Raven Press, New York, pp. 51–59.

Gulick, A., 1922, A study of weight regulation in the adult human body during overnutrition. *Amer. J. Physiol., 60,* 371–395.

Gwinup, G., 1975, Effect of exercise alone on the weight of obese women. *Arch. intern. Med., 135,* 676–680.

Hall, B., 1975, Changing composition of human milk and early development of appetite control. *Lancet, i,* 779–781.

Hall, S.M., Hall, R.G., DeBoer, G. and O'Kulitch, P., 1977, Self and external management compared with psychotherapy in the control of obesity. *Behav. Res. Ther., 15,* 89–95.

Halliday, D., 1967, Chemical composition of the whole body and individual tissues of two Jamaican children whose death resulted primarily from malnutrition. *Clin. Sci., 33,* 365–370.

Halliday, D., 1971, An attempt to estimate total body fat and protein in malnourished children. *Brit. J. Nutr., 26,* 147–153.

Halliday, D. and McKeran, R.O., 1975, Measurement of muscle protein synthetic rate from serial muscle biopsies and total body protein turnover in man by continuous infusion of L-[α-^{15}N]lysine. *Clin. Sci. mol. Med., 49,* 581–590.

Halliday, D. and Miller, A.G., 1977, Precise measurement of total body water using trace quantities of deuterium oxide. *Biomed. Mass Spectrom., 4,* 82–87.

Halliday, D., Hesp, R., Stalley, S.F., Warwick, P.M., Altman, D.G. and Garrow, J.S., 1978, Resting metabolic rate, weight, surface area and body composition in obese women on a reducing diet. *Int. J. Obesity,* in press.

Harding, R.H. and Sen, R.N., 1970, Evaluation of total muscular activity by quantification of electromyograms, through a summing amplifier. *Med. biol. Engng, 8,* 343–356.

Harrison, R. and Harden, R.M., 1966, The long term value of fasting in the treatment of obesity. *Lancet, ii,* 1340–1342.

Hashim, S.A. and Van Itallie, P.B., 1965, Studies in normal and obese subjects with a monitored food dispensing service. *Ann. N.Y. Acad. Sci., 131,* 654–661.

Hawes, S.F., Albert, A., Healy, M.J.R. and Garrow, J.S., 1972, A comparison of soft-tissue radiography, reflected ultrasound, skinfold calipers and thigh circumference for estimating the thickness of fat overlying the iliac crest and greater trochanter. *Proc. Nutr. Soc., 31,* 91A.

210

Hawkins, C., 1976, Anorexia and loss of weight. *Brit. med. J., 2*, 1373—1375.

Haymes, E.M., Lundegren, H.M., Loomis, J.L. and Buskirk, E.R., 1976, Validity of the ultrasonic technique as a method of measuring subcutaneous adipose tissue. *Ann. hum. Biol., 3*, 245—251.

Heaton, K.W., 1973, Food fibre as an obstacle to energy intake. *Lancet, ii*, 1418—1421.

Heber, K.R., 1975, Double-blind trial of mazindol in overweight patients. *Med. J. Aust., 2*, 566—567.

Hedenstierna, G. and Santesson, J., 1976, Breathing mechanics, dead space and gas exchange in the extremely obese breathing spontaneously and during anaesthesia with intermittent positive pressure ventilation. *Acta anaesth. scand., 20*, 248—254.

Herman, C.P. and Mack, D., 1975, Restrained and unrestrained eating. *J. Personality, 43*, 647—660.

Herman, C.P. and Polivy, J., 1975, Anxiety, restraint and eating behaviour. *J. abnorm. Psychol., 84*, 666—672.

Hermann, L.S. and Iverson, M., 1968, Death during therapeutic starvation. *Lancet, ii*, 217.

Hermansen, L. and Von Döbeln, W., 1971, Body fat and skinfold measurements. *Scand. J. clin. Lab. Invest., 27*, 315—319.

Hermreck, A.S., Jewell, W.R. and Hardin, C.S., 1976, Gastric bypass for morbid obesity. Results and complications. *Surgery, 80*, 498—505.

Hervey, G.R., 1969, Regulation of energy balance. *Nature (Lond.), 222*, 629—631.

Hibscher, J.A. and Herman, C.P., 1977, Obesity, dieting and the expression of "obese" characteristics. *J. comp. physiol. Psychol., 91*, 374—385.

Hill, G.L., Bradley, J.A., Collins, J.P., McCarthy, I., Oxby, C.B. and Burkinshaw, L., 1978, Fat-free body mass from skinfold thickness: a close relationship with total body nitrogen. *Brit. J. Nutr., 39*, 403—405.

Hirsch, J., 1975, Cell number and size as a determinant of subsequent obesity. In: M. Winick (Ed.), *Childhood Obesity*, Wiley, New York, pp. 15—21.

Hirsch, J. and Batchelor, B., 1976, Adipose tissue cellularity in human obesity. *Clin. endocr. Metab., 5*, 299—311.

Hirsch, J. and Gallian, E., 1968, Methods for the determination of adipose cell size in man and animals. *J. Lipid Res., 9*, 110—119.

Hirsch, J. and Goldrick, R.B., 1964, Serial studies on the metabolism of human adipose tissue. *J. clin. Invest., 43*, 1776—1792.

Hornberger, H.R., 1976, Gastric bypass. *Amer. J. Surg., 131*, 415—418.

Howard, A. and McLean Baird, I., 1977, A long-term evaluation of very low calorie semi-synthetic diets: an inpatient/outpatient study with egg albumin as the protein source. *Int. J. Obesity, 1*, 63—78.

Hultman, E., 1967, Muscle glycogen in man determined in needle biopsy specimens. *Scand. J. clin. Lab. Invest., 19*, 209—217.

Hunt, J.N., Cash, R. and Newland, P., 1975, Energy density of food, gastric emptying and obesity. *Lancet, ii*, 905—906.

Hytten, F.E., Taylor, K. and Taggart, N., 1966, Measurement of total body fat in man by absorption of [85]Kr. *Clin. Sci., 31*, 111—119.

Innes, J.A., Campbell, I.W., Campbell, C.J., Needle, A.L. and Munro, J.F., 1974,

Long-term follow up of therapeutic starvation. *Brit. med. J., 2*, 356.

Irsigler, K., Heitkamp, H., Schlick, W. and Schmid, P., 1975, Diet and energy balance in obesity. In: E. Jequier (Ed.), *Regulation of Energy Balance in Man*, Éditions Médecine et Hygiène, Geneva, pp. 72–83.

James, W.P.T. and Trayhurn, P., 1976, An integrated view of the metabolic and genetic basis for obesity. *Lancet, ii*, 770–772.

Jeejeebhoy, K.N., 1976, Total parenteral nutrition. *Ann. roy. Coll. Phycns Canada, 9*, 287–300.

Jéquier, E., Gygax, P.-H., Pittet, Ph. and Vanotti, A., 1974, Increased thermal body insulation: relationship to the development of obesity. *J. appl. Physiol., 36*, 674–678.

Johnson, S.F., Swenson, W.M. and Gastineau, C.F., 1976, Personality characteristics in obesity: relation to MMPI profile and age of onset of obesity to success in weight reduction. *Amer. J. clin. Nutr., 29*, 626–632.

Jolliffe, N. and Alpert, E., 1951, The 'performance index' as a method for estimating effectiveness of reducing regimens. *Postgrad. Med., 9*, 106–115.

Jones, P.R.M., Bharadwaj, H., Bhatia, M.R. and Malhotra, M.S., 1976, Differences between ethnic groups in the relationship of skinfold thickness to body density. In: B. Bhatia, G.S. Chhina and B. Singh (Eds.), *Selected Topics in Environmental Biology*, Interprint Publications, New Delhi, pp. 373–376.

Jourdan, M., Margen, S. and Bradfield, R.B., 1974, Protein-sparing effects in obese women fed low calorie diets. *Amer. J. clin. Nutr., 27*, 3–12.

Juhl, E., Bruusgaard, A., Hippe, E., Korner, B., Quaade, F. and Baden, H., 1974, Vitamin B_{12} depletion in obese patients treated with jejunoileal shunt. *Scand. J. Gastroenterol., 9*, 543–547.

Kairento, A.-L. and Spring, E., 1974, Measurement of bone mineral and body composition by the attenuation of three low energy radiation from [241]Am. *Ann. clin. Res., 6*, 80–85.

Kalucy, R.S., Crisp, A.H., Chard, T., McNeilly, A., Chen, C.N. and Lacey, J.H., 1976, Nocturnal hormonal profiles in massive obesity, anorexia nervosa and normal females. *J. psychosom. Res., 20*, 595–604.

Kaplan, M.L. and Leveille, G.A., 1976, Calorigenic responses in obese and non-obese women. *Amer. J. clin. Nutr., 29*, 1108–1113.

Kasper, H., Schönborn, J. and Rabast, U., 1975, Behaviour of body weight under a low carbohydrate, high fat diet. *Amer. J. clin. Nutr., 28*, 800–801.

Kavanagh, M., 1972, Food sharing behaviour within a group of Douc monkeys. *Nature (Lond.), 239*, 406–407.

Kempner, W., Newborg, B.C., Peschel, R.L. and Skyler, J.S., 1975, Treatment of massive obesity with rice/reduction diet programme. *Arch. intern. Med., 135*, 1575–1584.

Kennedy, G.C., 1950, The hypothalamic control of food intake in rats. *Proc. roy. Soc. B, 137*, 535–549.

Kennedy, G.C., 1953, The role of depot fat in the hypothalamic control of food intake in the rat. *Proc. roy. Soc. B, 140*, 578–596.

Kennedy, G.C., 1966, Food intake, energy balance and growth. *Brit. med. Bull., 22*, 216–220.

212

Keys, A. and Brozek, J., 1953, Body fat in adult man. *Physiol. Rev., 33*, 245– 325.

Keys, A., Brozek, J., Hanschel, A., Mickelson, O. and Taylor, H.L., 1950, *The Biology of Human Starvation*, University of Minnesota Press, Minneapolis, Minn., 1385 pp.

Keys, A., Aravanis, C., Blackburn, H., Buchem, F.S.P., Buzina, R., Djordjevic, B.S., Fidansa, F., Karvonen, M.J., Menotti, V. and Taylor, H.L., 1972, Coronary heart disease: overweight and obesity as risk factors. *Ann. intern. Med., 77*, 15–27.

Khosla, T. and Billewicz, W.Z., 1964, Measurement of change of body weight. *Brit. J. Nutr., 18*, 227–239.

Khosla, T. and Lowe, C.R., 1971, Obesity and smoking habits. *Brit. med. J., 4*, 10–13.

Khosla, T. and Lowe, C.R., 1972, Obesity and smoking habits by social class. *Brit. J. prev. soc. Med., 26*, 249–256.

Kihlström, J.E. and Lundberg, C., 1971, Cyclical variations of body temperatures in female rabbits before and after ovariectomy. *Acta physiol. scand., 82*, 272–276.

Kirby, M. and Turner, P., 1976, Hypothesis. Do "anorectic" drugs produce weight loss by appetite suppression? *Lancet, i*, 566–567.

Kirtland, J., Gurr, M.I., Saville, G. and Widdowson, E.M., 1975, Occurrence of "pockets" of very small cells in adipose tissue of the guinea pig. *Nature (Lond.), 256*, 723–724.

Kjelberg, J., Levi, L., Palmblad, J., Paulsson, L., Theorell, T. and Yensen, R., 1977, Energy deprivation in man – methodological problems and possibilities. *Acta med. scand., 201*, 9–13.

Knittle, J.L., Ginsberg-Fellner, F. and Brown, R.E., 1977, Adipose tissue development in man. *Amer. J. clin. Nutr., 30*, 762–766.

Kodama, A.M., Pace, N. and Pavot, S.J., 1974, Accuracy of measurement of potassium content of monkeys by in vivo body counting as compared with chemical analysis. *Phys. Biol. Med., 19*, 862–873.

Kofranyi, E. and Michaelis, H.F., 1940, Ein tragbarer Apparat zur Bestimmung des Gasstoffwechsels. *Arbeitsphysiologie, 11*, 148–150.

Krebs, H.A., 1964, The metabolic fate of amino acids. In: H.N. Munro and J.B. Allison (Eds.), *Mammalian Protein Metabolism*, Academic Press, New York, pp. 125–176.

Krotkiewski, M., Sjöström, L., Björntorp, P., Carlgren, G., Garellick, G. and Smith, U., 1977, Adipose tissue cellularity in relation to prognosis for weight reduction. *Int. J. Obesity, 1*, 395–416.

Landis, C., 1925, Studies of emotional reactions. IV. Metabolic rate. *Amer. J. Physiol., 74*, 188–203.

Lawrence, J.S., 1975, Hypertension in relation to musculoskeletal diseases. *Ann. rheum. Dis., 34*, 451–456.

Leach, R.E., Baumgard, S. and Broom, J., 1973, Obesity: its relationship to osteoarthritis of the knee. *Clin. Orthop., 93*, 271–273.

Leelartheapin, B., Woodhill, J.M., Palmer, A.J. and Blacket, R.B., 1974, Obesity, diet and type II hyperlipidaemia. *Lancet, ii*, 1217–1221.

Leibling, D.S., Eisner, J.D., Gibbs, J. and Smith, G.P., 1975, Intestinal satiety in rats. *J. comp. physiol. Psychol., 89*, 955–965.

Lesser, G.T., Deutsch, S. and Markofsky, J., 1971, Use of independent measurement of body fat to evaluate overweight and underweight. *Metabolism, 20*, 792–804.

Lewis, S., Haskell, W.L., Klein, H., Halpern, J. and Wood, P.D., 1975, Prediction of body composition in habitually active middle-aged men. *J. appl. Physiol., 39*, 221–225.

Lewis, S., Haskell, W.L., Wood, P.D., Manoogian, N., Bailey, J.E. and Pereira, M.B., 1976, Effects of physical activity on weight reduction in obese middle-aged women. *Amer. J. clin. Nutr., 29*, 151–156.

Ley, P., Bradshaw, P.W., Kincey, J.A., Couper-Smartt, J. and Wilson, M., 1974, Psychological variables in the control of obesity. In: W.L. Burland, P. Samuel and J. Yudin (Eds.), *Obesity*, Churchill-Livingstone, Edinburgh, pp. 316–337.

Lincoln, J.E., 1972, Calorie intake, obesity and physical activity. *Amer. J. clin. Nutr., 25*, 390–394.

Lindstrom, L.L., Balch, P. and Reese, S., 1976, In person versus telephone treatment for obesity. *J. behav. Ther. exp. Psychiat., 7*, 367–369.

Lipner, A., 1977, Symptomatic magnesium deficiency after small-intestinal bypass for obesity. *Brit. med. J., 1*, 148.

Loffer, F.E. and Pent, D., 1976, Laparoscopy in the obese patient. *Amer. J. Obstet. Gynec., 125*, 104–107.

Maagøe, H. and Mogensen, E.F., 1970, Effect of treatment on obesity: a follow-up of material treated with complete starvation. *Dan. med. Bull., 17*, 206–209.

MacCuish, A.C., Munro, J.F. and Duncan, L.J.P., 1968, Follow-up study of refractory obesity treated by fasting. *Brit. med. J., 1*, 91–92.

Mackarness, R., 1958, *Eat Fat and Grow Slim*, Harvill Press, London, 128 pp.

Maclay, W.P. and Wallace, M.G., 1977, A multi-centre general practice trial of mazindol in the treatment of obesity. *Practitioner, 218*, 431–434.

Maeder, E.C., Barno, A. and Mecklenburg, F., 1975, Obesity: a maternal high risk factor. *Obstet. and Gynec., 45*, 669–671.

Mahadeva, K., Passmore, R. and Woolf, B., 1953, Individual variations in metabolic cost of standardised exercises: effects of food, age, sex and race. *J. Physiol. (Lond.), 121*, 225–231.

Mahler, R., 1972, The relationship between eating and obesity. *Acta diabet. lat., 9*, 449–465.

Mann, G.V., Teel, K., Hayes, O., McNally, A. and Bruno, D., 1955, Exercise in the disposition of dietary calories: regulation of serum lipoprotein and cholesterol in human subjects. *New Engl. J. Med., 253*, 349–355.

Marr, J.W., 1971, Individual dietary surveys: purposes and methods. *Wld Rev. Nutr. Diet., 13*, 105–164.

Martineaud, M. and Trémolière, J., 1964, Mesures de la dépense calorique basale dans l'obésité. *Nutr. et Dieta (Basel), 6*, 77–85.

Mason, E.E. and Ito, C., 1969, Gastric bypass. *Ann. Surg., 170*, 329–336.

Mayer, J., 1952, Food composition tables and assessment of the caloric content of diets. *J. Amer. diet. Ass., 28*, 308–312.

Mayer, J., 1953, Genetic, traumatic and environmental factors in the aetiology of obesity. *Physiol. Rev., 33,* 472–508.

Mayer, J., 1970, Some aspects of the problem of regulating food intake and obesity. In: C.V. Rowland (Ed.), *Anorexia and Obesity, Vol. 7,* Little, Brown and Co., Boston, Mass., pp. 255–334.

Mayer, J. and Arees, E.A., 1968, Ventromedial glucoreceptor system. *Fed. Proc., 27,* 1345–1348.

Mayer, J., Roy, P. and Mitra, K.P., 1956, Relation between caloric intake, body weight and physical work: studies in an industrial male population in West Bengal. *Amer. J. clin. Nutr., 4,* 169–175.

McCance, R.A. and Widdowson, E.M., 1951, A method of breaking down the body weights of living persons into terms of extracellular fluid, cell mass and fat, and some applications of it to physiology and medicine. *Proc. roy. Soc. B, 138,* 115–130.

McCance, R.A. and Widdowson, E.M., 1960, *The Composition of Foods,* Medical Research Council, Spec. Rep. Ser. 297 (3rd ed.), H.M.S.O., London, 270 pp.

McCarthy, M.C., 1966, Dietary and activity patterns of obese women in Trinidad. *J. Amer. diet. Ass., 48,* 33–37.

McIntosh, J.F., Moller, E. and Van Slyke, D.D., 1929, Studies of urea excretion. III. The influence of body size on urea output. *J. clin. Invest., 6,* 467–483.

Mellbin, T. and Vuille, J.-C., 1973, Physical development at 7 years in relation to velocity of weight gain in infancy with special reference to incidence of overweight. *Brit. J. prev. soc. Med., 27,* 225–235.

Merimee, T.J. and Fineberg, E.S., 1976, Starvation-induced alterations of circulating thyroid hormone concentrations in man. *Metabolism, 25,* 79–83.

Metzner, H.L., Lamphiear, D.E., Wheeler, N.C. and Larkin, F.A., 1977, Relationship between frequency of eating and adiposity in adult men and women in the Tecumseh Community Health Study. *Amer. J. clin. Nutr., 30,* 712–715.

Millard, R.J., 1977, How much intravenous fluid does the patient get? *Lancet, ii,* 665–666.

Miller, D.S. and Mumford, P., 1967, Gluttony. 1. An experimental study of overeating on low or high protein diets. *Amer. J. clin. Nutr., 20,* 1212–1222.

Miller, D.S. and Parsonage, S., 1975, Resistance to slimming. Adaptation or illusion? *Lancet, i,* 773–775.

Miller, D.S., Mumford, P. and Stock, M.J., 1967, Gluttony. 2. Thermogenesis in over-eating man. *Amer. J. clin. Nutr., 20,* 1223–1229.

Mitchell, H.H., Hamilton, T.S., Steggerda, F.R. and Bean, H.W., 1945, The chemical composition of the adult human body and its bearing on the biochemistry of growth. *J. biol. Chem., 158,* 625–637.

Montoye, H.J., Epstein, F.H. and Kjelsberg, M.O., 1965, The measurement of body fatness: a study in a total community. *Amer. J. clin. Nutr., 16,* 417–427.

Morin, R.J. and Barry, R.E., 1976, Lipid composition of bile in morbid obesity before and after jejunoileal bypass surgery. *Clin. chim. Acta, 69,* 479–489.

Morris, J.N., Marr, J.W. and Clayton, D.G., 1977, Diet and heart: a postscript. *Brit. med. J., 2,* 1307–1314.

Morrow, C.P., Hernandez, W.L., Townsend, D.E. and Disaia, P.J., 1977, Pelvic celiotomy in the obese patient. *Amer. J. Obstet. Gynec., 127*, 335–339.

Morse, W.I. and Soeldner, J.S., 1963, The composition of adipose tissue and the non-adipose body of obese and non-obese man. *Metabolism, 12*, 99–107.

Moss, A.J. and Wynar, B., 1970, Tachycardia in house officers presenting cases at grand rounds. *Ann. intern. Med., 72*, 255–256.

Mulcare, D.B., Dennin, H.F. and Drenick, E.J., 1970, Effect of diet on malabsorption after small bowel bypass. *J. Amer. diet. Ass., 57*, 331–334.

Munro, J.F., MacCuish, A.C., Wilson, E.M. and Duncan, L.J.P., 1968, Comparison of continuous and intermittent anorectic therapy in obesity. *Brit. med. J., 1*, 352–354.

Munro, J.F., MacCuish, A.C., Goodall, J.A.D., Fraser, J. and Duncan, L.J.P., 1970, Further experience with prolonged therapeutic starvation in gross refractory obesity. *Brit. med. J.*, 712–714.

Nadal, R., Nel, M. and Ravina, A., 1954, Obésité et roentgen thérapie hypophysaire. *Presse méd., 62*, 1664–1667.

Neshat, A.A. and Flye, M.W., 1975, Early formation of gallstones following jejunoileal bypass for treatment of morbid obesity. *Amer. Surg., 41*, 486–491.

Neumann, R.O., 1902, Experimentelle Beiträge zur Lehre von dem täglichen Nahrungsbedarf des Menschen unter besonderer Berücksichtigung der notwendigen Eiweissmenge. *Arch. Hyg. (Berl.), 45*, 1.

Nicoloff, J.T., Low, J.C., Dessault, J.H. and Fisher, D.A., 1972, Simultaneous measurement of thyroxine and triiodothyronine peripheral turnover kinetics in man. *J. clin. Invest., 51*, 473–483.

Nielsen, W.C., Krzywicki, H.J., Honson, H.L. and Consolazio, C.F., 1971, Use and evaluation of gas chromatography for determination of deuterium in body fluids. *J. appl. Physiol., 31*, 957–961.

Nisbett, R.E., 1968, Determinants of food intake in obesity. *Science, 159*, 1254–1255.

Nishizawa, T., Akaoka, I., Nishida, Y., Kawaguchi, Y., Hayashi, E. and Yoshimura, T., 1976, Some factors related to obesity in the Japanese sumo wrestler. *Amer. J. clin. Nutr., 29*, 1167–1174.

Norbury, F.B., 1964, Contraindications to long-term fasting. *J. Amer. med. Ass., 188*, 88.

Olsson, K.-E. and Saltin, B., 1970, Variation in total body water with muscle glycogen in man. *Acta physiol. scand., 80*, 11–18.

Orsini, D. and Passmore, R., 1951, The energy expended carrying loads up and down stairs: experiments using the Kofranyi–Michaelis calorimeter. *J. Physiol. (Lond.), 115*, 95–100.

Ounstead, M. and Sleigh, G., 1975, The infant's self-regulation of food intake and weight gain. *Lancet, i*, 1393–1397.

Pace, N. and Rathbun, E.N., 1945, Studies on body composition. III. Water and chemically contained nitrogen content in relation to fat content. *J. biol. Chem., 158*, 685–691.

Palmblad, J., Levi, L., Burger, A., Melander, A., Westgren, U., Von Schenk, H. and Skude, G., 1977, Effects of total energy withdrawal (fasting) on the levels of growth hormone, thyrotropin, cortisol, adrenaline, noradrenaline, T_4, T_3 and rT_3 in healthy males. *Acta med. scand., 201,* 15–22.

Palmquist, D.L., Learn, D.B. and Baker, N., 1977, Re-evaluation of effects of meal feeding on lipogenic activation by glucose in rats. *J. Nutr., 107,* 502–509.

Parnell, R.W., 1977, How dangerous is obesity? *Brit. med. J., 1,* 1345–1346.

Passmore, R., 1967, Energy balances in man. *Proc. Nutr. Soc., 26,* 97–101.

Passmore, R. and Durnin, J.V.G.A., 1955, Human energy expenditure. *Physiol. Rev., 35,* 801–840.

Passmore, R., Thomson, J.G. and Warnock, G.M., 1952, A balance sheet of the estimation of energy intake and energy expenditure as measured by indirect calorimetry using the Kofranyi–Michaelis calorimeter. *Brit. J. Nutr., 6,* 253–264.

Passmore, R., Meiklejohn, A.P., Dewar, A.D. and Thow, R.K., 1955a, Energy utilization in overfed thin men. *Brit. J. Nutr., 9,* 20–26.

Passmore, R., Meiklejohn, A.P., Dewar, A.D. and Thow, R.K., 1955b, An analysis of the gain in weight of overfed thin young men. *Brit. J. Nutr., 9,* 27–37.

Passmore, R., Strong, J.A. and Ritchie, F.J., 1958, The chemical composition of the tissue lost by obese patients on a reducing regimen. *Brit. J. Nutr., 12,* 113–122.

Passmore, R., Strong, J.A., Swindells, Y.E. and El Din, N., 1963, The effect of overfeeding on two fat young women. *Brit. J. Nutr., 17,* 373–383.

Paul, D.R., Hoyt, J.L. and Boutros, A.R., 1976, Cardiovascular and respiratory changes in response to change of posture in the very obese. *Anaesthesia, 45,* 73–78.

Paulsen, B.K., Lutz, R.N., McReynolds, W.T. and Kohrs, M.B., 1976, Behaviour therapy for weight control: long term results of two programs with nutritionists as therapists. *Amer. J. clin. Nutr., 29,* 880–888.

Pavel, I., Sdrobici, D. and Dumitrescu, C., 1969, The long term efficiency of weight reducing curves for obesity. *Rum. med. Rev., 13,* 14–22.

Pawan, G.L.S. and Clode, M., 1960, The gross chemical composition of subcutaneous adipose tissue in the lean and obese human subject. *Biochem. J., 74,* 9P.

Paykel, E.S., Mueller, P.S. and De la Vergne, P.M., 1973, Amitryptyline, weight gain and carbohydrate craving: a side effect. *Brit. J. Psychiat., 123,* 501–507.

Payne, P.R. and Dugdale, A.E., 1977, Mechanism for the control of body-weight. *Lancet, i,* 583–586.

Pearson, D., 1970, *The Chemical Analysis of Food,* 6th ed., Churchill, London, p. 16.

Peckham, C.H. and Christianson, R.E., 1971, The relationship between prepregnancy weight and certain obstetric factors. *Amer. J. Obstet. Gynec., 111,* 1–7.

Pelkonen, R., Nikkila, E., Koskinen, S., Penttinen, K. and Sarna, S., 1977, Association of serum lipids and obesity with cardiovascular mortality. *Brit. med. J., 2,* 1185–1187.

Pequignot, G., Vinit, F., Richard, J.L., Cubeau, J., Papoz, L. and Laquerriere, A.,

1973, Absence of relation between stoutness and food intake. In: M. Apfelbaum (Ed.), *Energy Balance in Man*, Masson, Paris, pp. 61–64.

Peto, R. and Doll, R., 1977, When is significant not significant? *Brit. med. J., 2*, 259.

Pflanz, M., 1962, Medizinisch-soziologische Aspekte der Fettsucht. *Psyche, 16*, 575–591.

Pierson, R.N., Wang, J., Yang, M.U., Hashim, S.A. and Van Itallie, T.B., 1976, The assessment of body composition during weight reduction: evaluation of a new model for clinical studies. *J. Nutr., 106*, 1694–1701.

Pilkington, T.R.E., Gazet, J.-C., Ang, L., Kalucy, R.S., Crisp, A.H. and Day, S., 1976, Explanation for weight loss after ileojejunal bypass in gross obesity. *Brit. med. J., 1*, 1504–1505.

Pittet, Ph., Chappuis, Ph., Acheson, K., De Techtermann, F. and Jéquier, E., 1976, Thermic effect of glucose in obese subjects studied by direct and indirect calorimetry. *Brit. J. Nutr., 35*, 281–292.

Pollock, M.L., Loughridge, E.E., Coleman, B., Limerud, A.C. and Jackson, A., 1975, Prediction of body density in young and middle-aged women. *J. appl. Physiol., 38*, 745–749.

Poskitt, E.M.E. and Cole, T.J., 1977, Do fat babies stay fat? *Brit. med. J., 1*, 7–9.

Pozefsky, T., Tancredi, R.G., Moxley, R.T., Dupre, J. and Tobin, J.D., 1976, Effects of brief starvation on muscle amino acid metabolism in nonobese man. *J. clin. Invest., 57*, 444–449.

Preece, P.E., Richards, A.R., Owen, G.M. and Hughes, L.E., 1975, Mastalgia and total body water. *Brit. med. J., 4*, 498–500.

Premachandra, B.N. and Perlstein, I.B., 1976, Studies on obesity. III. Effect of triiodothyronine (T_3) on thyroglobulin autoantibodies in euthyroid obese subjects. *Metabolism, 25*, 981–988.

Printen, K.H. and Mason, E.E., 1977, Gastric bypass for morbid obesity in patients more than fifty years of age. *Surg. Gynec. Obstet., 144*, 192–194.

Pudel, V.E. and Oetting, M., 1977, Eating in the laboratory: behavioural aspects of the positive energy balance. *Int. J. Obesity, 1*, 369–386.

Quaade, F., 1963, Insulation in leanness and obesity. *Lancet, ii*, 429–432.

Quaade, F., 1974, Stereotaxy for obesity. *Lancet, i*, 267.

Ravelli, G.-O., Stein, Z.A. and Susser, M.W., 1976, Obesity in young men after famine exposure in utero and early infancy. *New Engl. J. Med., 295*, 349–353.

Reed, R.B. and Burke, B.S., 1954, Collection and analysis of dietary intake data. *Amer. J. publ. Hlth, 44*, 1015–1026.

Reuben, D., 1976, *The Save your Life Diet*, Ebury Press, London, 160 pp.

Ries, W., 1973, Feeding behaviour in obesity. *Proc. Nutr. Soc., 32*, 187–193.

Rimm, I.J. and Rimm, A.A., 1976, Association between juvenile onset obesity and severe adult obesity in 73,532 women. *Amer. J. publ. Hlth, 66*, 479–481.

Rimm, A., Werner, L.H., Van Yserloo, B. and Bernstein, R.A., 1975, Relationship of obesity to disease in 73,522 weight conscious women. *Publ. Hlth Rep., 90*, 44–52.

218

Robinson, M.F. and Watson, P.E., 1965, Day-to-day variations in body weight of young women. *Brit. J. Nutr., 19*, 225–235.

Rochelle, R.H. and Horvath, S.M., 1969, Metabolic responses to food and acute cold stress. *J. appl. Physiol., 27*, 710–714.

Rodgers, S., Burnet, R., Goss, A., Phillips, P., Goldney, R., Kimber, C., Thomas, D., Harding, P. and Wise, P., 1977, Jaw wiring in the treatment of obesity. *Lancet, i*, 1221–1223.

Rodin, J., 1975, Effects of obesity and set point on taste responsiveness and ingestion in humans. *J. comp. physiol. Psychol., 89*, 1003–1009.

Rodin, J., Bray, G.A., Atkinson, R.L., Dahms, W.T., Greenway, F.L., Hamilton, K. and Molitch, M., 1977a, Predictors of successful weight loss in an outpatient clinic. *Int. J. Obesity, 1*, 79–87.

Rodin, J., Slochower, J. and Fleming, B., 1977b, Effects of degree of obesity, age of onset, and weight loss on responsiveness to sensory and external stimuli. *J. comp. physiol. Psychol., 91*, 586–597.

Rooth, G. and Carlström, S., 1970, Therapeutic fasting. *Acta med. scand., 187*, 455–463.

Ross, M.H. and Bras, G., 1975, Food preference and length of life. *Science, 190*, 165–167.

Ross, M.H., Lustbader, E. and Bras, G., 1976, Dietary practices as predictors of longevity. *Nature (Lond.), 262*, 548–553.

Rozin, P., 1976, Psychobiological and cultural determinants of food choice. In: T. Silverstone (Ed.), *Appetite and Food Intake*, Dahlem Konferenzen, Berlin, pp. 285–312.

Ruiz, L., Colley, J.R.T. and Hamilton, P.J.S., 1971, Measurement of triceps skinfold thickness. An investigation of sources of variation. *Brit. J. prev. soc. Med., 25*, 165–167.

Runcie, J. and Hilditch, T.E., 1974, Energy provision, tissue utilization and weight loss in prolonged starvation. *Brit. med. J., 2*, 352–356.

Runcie, J. and Thomson, T.J., 1970, Prolonged starvation: a dangerous procedure? *Brit. med. J., 3*, 432–435.

Russek, M., 1976, A conceptual equation of intake control. In: D. Novin, W. Wyrwicka and G. Bray (Eds.), *Hunger: Basic Mechanisms and Clinical Implications,* Raven Press, New York, pp. 327–347.

Sanders, M. and Breidahl, H., 1976, The effects of an anorectic agent (Mazindol) on control of obese diabetics. *Med. J. Aust., 2*, 576–577.

Saraiva, R.A., Lunn, J.N., Mapleson, W.W., Willis, B.A. and France, J.M., 1977, Adiposity and the pharmacokinetics of halothane. The effect of adiposity on the maintenance of and recovery from halothane anaesthesia. *Anaesthesia, 32*, 240–246.

Sash, S.E., 1977, Why is the treatment of obesity a failure in modern society? *Int. J. Obesity, 1*, 247–248.

Schachter, S., 1968, Obesity and eating: internal and external cues differentially affect the eating behaviour of obese and normal subjects. *Science, 161*, 751–756.

Schmid, P., Schlick, W. and Irsigler, K., 1974, Is there retention or production of nitrogen or other gases except O_2 and CO_2 in human steady state conditions? *Metabolism, 23*, 703–708.

Scott, W.H., Brill, A.B. and Price, R.R., 1975, Body composition in morbidly obese patients before and after jejunoileal bypass. *Ann. Surg., 182*, 395–404.

Seltzer, C.C. and Mayer, J., 1965, A simple criterion of obesity. *Postgrad. Med., 38A*, 101–107.

Shapiro, B., 1973, Regulation of adipose tissue size. In: M. Apfelbaum (Ed.), *Energy Balance in Man*, Masson, Paris, pp. 247–259.

Sharma, B., Thadani, U. and Taylor, S.H., 1974, Cardiovascular effects of weight reduction in obese patients with angina pectoris. *Brit. Heart J., 36*, 854–858.

Shearer, R.S. and Keily, J.J., 1977, New techniques for office management of obesity. *J. intern. Med. Res., 5*, 147–154.

Shephard, R.J., 1955, A critical examination of the Douglas bag technique. *J. Physiol. (Lond.), 127*, 515–524.

Shetty, K.R. and Kalkhoff, R.K., 1977, Human chorionic gonadotrophic (HCG) treatment of obesity. *Arch. intern. Med., 137*, 151–155.

Shizgal, H.M., 1976, Total body potassium and nutritional status. *Surg. Clin. N. Amer., 56*, 1185–1194.

Silverstone, T., 1975, Anorectic drugs. In: T. Silverstone (Ed.), *Obesity: Pathogenesis and Management*, M.T.P., Lancaster, pp. 193–227.

Silverstone, T. and Fincham, J., 1978, Techniques for the evaluation of anorectic drugs. In: S. Garattini and R. Samanin (Eds.), Central Actions of Anorectic Drugs, Raven Press, New York.

Silverstone, J.T., Stark, J.E. and Buckle, R.M., 1966, Hunger during total starvation. *Lancet, i*, 1343–1344.

Silverstone, J.T., Gordon, R.P. and Stunkard, A.J., 1969, Social factors in obesity in London. *Practitioner, 202*, 682–688.

Sims, E.A.H., Goldman, R.F., Gluck, C.M., Horton, E.S., Kelleher, P.C. and Rowe, D.W., 1968, Experimental obesity in man. *Trans. Ass. Amer. Phycns, 81*, 153–170.

Siri, W.E., 1961, Body volume measurement by gas dilution. In: J. Brozek and A. Henschel (Eds.), *Techniques for Measuring Body Composition*, National Academy of Sciences, Washington, D.C., pp. 180–217.

Sjöström, L., 1976, Comments on adipocyte sizing. *Clin. chim. Acta, 74*, 89–91.

Smith, R.G., Innes, J.A. and Munro, J.F., 1975, Double blind evaluation of Mazindol in refractory obesity. *Brit. med. J., 3*, 284.

Sohar, E., Scapa, E. and Ravid, M., 1973, Constancy of relative body weight in children. *Arch. Dis. Childh., 48*, 389–392.

Solow, C., Silberfarb, P.M. and Swift, K., 1974, Psychosocial effects of intestinal bypass surgery for severe obesity. *New Engl. J. Med., 290*, 300–304.

Soper, R.T., Mason, E.E., Printen, K.J. and Zellweger, H., 1975, Gastric bypass for morbid obesity in children and adolescents. *J. pediat. Surg., 10*, 51–58.

Sorensen, T.I.A. and Sonne-Holm, S., 1977, Mortality in extremely overweight young men. *J. chron. Dis., 30*, 359–367.

Southgate, D.A.T. and Durnin, J.V.G.A., 1970, Calorie conversion factors: an experimental reassessment of the factors used in the calculation of the energy value of human diets. *Brit. J. Nutr., 24*, 517–535.

Spady, D.W., Payne, P.R., Picou, D. and Waterlow, J.C., 1976, Energy balance during recovery from malnutrition. *Amer. J. clin. Nutr., 29*, 1073–1088.

Spainier, A.H. and Shizgal, H.M., 1977, Caloric requirements of the critically ill patient receiving intravenous hyperalimentation. *Amer. J. Surg., 133*, 99–104.

Spaulding, S.W., 1976, Effect of caloric restriction and dietary composition on serum T_3 and reverse T_3 in man. *J. clin. Endocr., 42*, 197–200.

Spencer, I.O.B., 1968, Death during therapeutic starvation for obesity. *Lancet, i*, 1288–1290.

Spiegel, T.A., 1973, Caloric regulation of food intake in man. *J. comp. physiol. Psychol., 84*, 24–37.

Spinnler, G., Jéquier, E., Favre, R., Dolivo, M. and Vanotti, A., 1973, Human calorimeter with a new type of gradient layer. *J. appl. Physiol., 35*, 158–165.

Steel, J.M. and Briggs, M., 1972, Withdrawal depression in obese patients after fenfluramine treatment. *Brit. med. J., 3*, 26–27.

Steel, J.M., Munro, J.F. and Duncan, L.J.P., 1973, A comparative trial of different regimens of fenfluramine and phentermine in obesity. *Practitioner, 211*, 232–236.

Stefanik, P.A., Heald, F.P. and Mayer, J., 1959, Calorie intake in relation to energy output of obese and non-obese adolescent boys. *Amer. J. clin. Nutr., 7*, 55–62.

Stein, M.R., Julis, R.E., Peck, C.C., Hinshaw, W., Sawicki, J.E. and Deller, J.J., 1976, Ineffectiveness of human chorionic gonadotropin in weight reduction: a double-blind study. *Amer. J. clin. Nutr., 29*, 940–948.

Steinkamp, R.C., Cohen, N.L., Gaffey, W.R., McKey, T., Bron, G., Siri, W.E., Saregent, T.W. and Isaacs, E., 1965, Measures of body fat and related factors in normal adults. II. A simple clinical method to estimate body fat and lean body mass. *J. chron. Dis., 18*, 1291–1307.

Stordy, B.J., Marks, V., Kalucy, R.S. and Crisp, A.H., 1977, Weight gain, thermic effect of glucose and resting metabolism rate during recovery from anorexia nervosa. *Amer. J. clin. Nutr., 30*, 138–146.

Strakova, M. and Markova, J., 1971, Ultrasound used for measuring subcutaneous fat. *Rev. Czeck. Med., 17*, 66–73.

Strong, J.A., Shirling, D. and Passmore, R., 1967, Some effects of overfeeding for four days in man. *Brit. J. Nutr., 21*, 909–919.

Stuart, R.B., 1967, Behavioural control of overeating. *Behav. Res. Ther., 5*, 357–365.

Stuart, R.B., 1976, Behavioural control of overeating: a status report. In: G. Bray (Ed.), *Obesity in Perspective*, Fogarty International Center, U.S. Government Printing Office, Washington, D.C., pp. 367–385.

Stunkard, A.J., 1972, New therapies for the eating disorders: behaviour modification of obesity and anorexia nervosa. *Arch. gen. Psychiat., 26*, 391–398.

Stunkard, A.J. and Fox, S., 1971, The relationship of gastric motility and hunger. *Psychosom. Med., 33*, 123–134.

Stunkard, A.J. and McLaren-Hume, M., 1959, The results of treatment for obesity. *Arch. intern. Med., 103*, 79–85.

Sullivan, L., 1976, Metabolic and physiologic effects of physical training in hyperplastic obesity. *Scand. J. rehab. Med., Suppl. 5*, 38 pp.

Swenson, S.A., Lewis, J.W. and Sebby, K.R., 1974, Magnesium metabolism in man with special reference to jejunoileal bypass for obesity. *Amer. J. Surg.,* *127,* 250–255.

Swift, R.W., Barron, G.P., Fisher, K.H., Magruder, N.D., Black, A., Bratzler, J.W., French, C.E., Hartsook, E.W., Hershberger, T.V., Keck, E. and Stiles, F.P., 1957, *Relative Dynamic Effects of High versus Low Protein Diets of Equicaloric Content*, Department of Animal Nutrition, Pennsylvania State University Publication No. 232.

Taggart, N., 1962, Diet, activity and body weight. A study of variations in a woman. *Brit. J. Nutr., 16,* 223–235.

Talbot, N.B., 1938, Measurement of obesity by the creatinine coefficient. *Amer. J. Dis. Child., 55,* 42–50.

Tanner, J.M., 1965, Radiographic studies of body composition in children and adults. In: J. Brozek (Ed.), *Human Body Composition*, Pergamon Press, Oxford, pp. 211–236.

Tata, J.R., 1964, Advances in metabolic disorders. In: R. Levine and R. Luft (Eds.), *Basal Metabolic Rate and Thyroid Hormones*, Academic Press, New York, pp. 153–189.

Tewksbury, D.A. and Lohrenz, F.N., 1970, Circadian rhythm of human urinary amino acid excretion in fed and fasted states. *Metabolism, 19,* 363–371.

Thomas, L.W., 1962, Chemical composition of adipose tissue of man and mice. *Quart. J. exp. Physiol., 47,* 179–188.

Thompson, D.A., Moskowitz, H.R. and Campbell, R.G., 1976, Effects of body weight and food intake on pleasantness ratings for a sweet stimulus. *J. appl. Physiol., 41,* 77–83.

Thomson, A.M., 1958, Diet in pregnancy. I. Diet survey technique and the nutritive value of diets taken by primigravidae. *Brit. J. Nutr., 12,* 446–461.

Thomson, A.M., Billewicz, W.Z. and Passmore, R., 1961, The relation between calorie intake and body weight in man. *Lancet, i,* 1027–1028.

Thomson, T.J., Runcie, J. and Miller, V., 1966, Treatment of obesity by total fasting up to 249 days. *Lancet, ii,* 992–996.

Trayhurn, P., Thurlby, P.L. and James, W.P.T., 1977, Thermogenic defect in pre-obese *ob/ob* mice. *Nature (Lond.), 266,* 60–62.

Trémolière, J., Carre, L. and Naon, R., 1973, Interrelations between body weight, level of vigilance and energy expenditure in subjects on various diets. In: M. Apfelbaum (Ed.), *Energy Balance in Man*, Masson, Paris, pp. 125–134.

Trulson, M.F., 1954, Assessment of dietary study methods. I. Comparison of methods for obtaining data for clinical work. *J. Amer. diet. Ass., 30,* 991–995.

Tullis, I.F., 1973, Rational diet for mild and grand obesity. *J. Amer. med. Ass., 226,* 70–73.

Turner, W.T. and Cohn, S., 1975, Total body potassium and 24 h creatinine excretion in healthy males. *Clin. Pharmacol. Ther., 18,* 405–412.

Underwood, P.J., Belton, E. and Hulme, P., 1973, Aversion to sucrose in obesity *Proc. Nutr. Soc., 32,* 92A–93A.

Unsigned Editorial, 1970, Thermogenesis. *Amer. J. clin. Nutr., 23,* 1009–1010.

Van den Berg, A.S. and Mayer, J., 1954, Comparison of a one-day food record and research dietary history on a group of obese pregnant women. *J. Amer. diet. Ass., 30,* 1239–1244.

222

Van Graan, C.H. and Wyndham, C.H., 1964, Body surface area in human beings. *Nature (Lond.)*, *204*, 998.

Van Itallie, T.B., Smith, N.S. and Quartermain, D., 1977, Short-term and long-term components in the regulation of food intake: evidence for a modulatory role of carbohydrate status. *Amer. J. clin. Nutr.*, *30*, 742–757.

Vaughan, R.W. and Wise, L., 1976, Intraoperative arterial oxygenation in obese patients. *Ann. Surg.*, *184*, 35–42.

Vaughan, R.W., Bauer, S. and Wise, L., 1975, Volume and pH of gastric juice in obese patients. *Anaesthesia*, *43*, 686–689.

Walike, B.C., Jordan, H.A. and Stellar, E., 1969, Preloading and the regulation of food intake in man. *J. comp. physiol. Psychol.*, *68*, 327–333.

Walker, B.R., Ballard, I.M. and Gold, J.A., 1977, A multicentre study comparing Mazindol and placebo in obese patients. *J. intern. Med. Res.*, *5*, 85–90.

Wang, J. and Pierson, R.N., 1976, Disparate hydration of adipose and lean tissue require a new model for body water distribution in man. *J. Nutr.*, *106*, 1687–1693.

Ward, G.M., Krzywicki, H.J., Rahman, D.P., Quaas, R.L., Nelson, R.A. and Consolazio, C.F., 1975, Relationship of anthropometric measurements of body fat as determined by densitometry, potassium[40] and body water. *Amer. J. clin. Nutr.*, *28*, 162–169.

Warnold, I. and Lenner, R.A., 1977, Evaluation of the heart rate method to determine the daily energy expenditure in disease. A study on juvenile diabetics. *Amer. J. clin. Nutr.*, *30*, 304–315.

Warwick, P.M., Toft, R. and Garrow, J.S., 1978, Individual variation in energy expenditure. In: G. Bray (Ed.), *Recent Advances in Obesity Research*, *Vol. 2,* Newman, London, in press.

Webb, P., Annis, J.F. and Troutman, S.J., 1972, Human calorimetry with a water-cooled garment. *J. appl. Physiol.*, *32*, 412–418.

Weir, J.B. de V., 1949, New methods for calculating metabolic rate with special reference to protein metabolism. *J. Physiol. (Lond.)*, *109*, 1–9.

Weinsier, R.L., Fuchs, R.J., Kay, T.D., Triebwasser, J.H. and Lancaster, M.C., 1976, Body fat: its relationship to coronary heart disease, blood pressure, lipids and other risk factors measured in a large male population. *Amer. J. Med.*, *61*, 815–824.

Weisenberg, M. and Frey, E., 1974, What's missing in the treatment of obesity by behaviour modification? *J. Amer. diet. Ass.*, *65*, 410–414.

Whipp, B.J., Bray, G. and Koyal, S.N., 1973, Exercise energetics in normal man following acute weight gain. *Amer. J. clin. Nutr.*, *26*, 1284–1286.

Whitelaw, A., 1977, Infant feeding and subcutaneous fat at birth and at one year. *Lancet*, *ii*, 1098–1099.

Widdowson, E.M., 1936, A study of English diets by the individual method. Part I. Men. *J. Hyg. (Lond.)*, *36*, 269–292.

Widdowson, E.M. and Dickerson, J.W.T., 1960, The effect of growth and function on the chemical composition of soft tissues. *Biochem. J.*, *77*, 30–43.

Widdowson, E.M., McCance, R.A. and Spray, C.M., 1951, The chemical composition of the human body. *Clin. Sci.*, *10*, 113–125.

Wilkinson, P.W., 1977, Energy intake and physical activity in obese children. *Brit. med. J.*, *1*, 756.

Wilkinson, P.W., Parkin, J.M., Pearlson, J., Philips, P.R. and Sykes, P., 1977, Obesity in childhood: a community study in Newcastle upon Tyne. *Lancet, i*, 350–352.

Wolff, H.S., 1956, Modern techniques for estimating energy expenditure. *Proc. Nutr. Soc., 15*, 77–80.

Wolgin, D.L., Cytawa, J. and Teitelbaum, P., 1976, The role of activation in the regulation of food intake. In: D. Novin, W. Wyrwicka and G.A. Bray (Eds.), *Hunger, Basic Mechanisms and Clinical Implications*, Raven Press, New York, pp. 179–191.

Womersley, J. and Durnin, J.V.G.A., 1977, A comparison of the skinfold method with extent of "overweight" and various weight-height relationships in the assessment of obesity. *Brit. J. Nutr., 38*, 271–284.

Womersley, J., Durnin, J.V.G.A., Boddy, K. and Mahaffy, M., 1976, Influence of muscular development, obesity and age on the fat-free mass of adults. *J. appl. Physiol., 41*, 223–229.

Wood, G.D., 1977, The early results of treatment of the obese by a diet regimen enforced by maxillomandibular fixation. *J. oral Surg., 35*, 461–464.

Woodward, E.R., Payne, J.H., Salmon, P.A. and O'Leary, J.P., 1976, A panel by correspondence: morbid obesity. *Arch. Surg., 110*, 1440–1445.

Wooley, O.W., 1971, Long-term food regulation in the obese and nonobese. *Psychosom. Med., 33*, 436–444.

Wooley, O.W., Wooley, S.C. and Dunham, R.B., 1972, Can calories be perceived and do they affect hunger in obese and non-obese humans? *J. comp. physiol. Psychol., 80*, 250–258.

Wooley, O.W., Wooley, S.C. and Dunham, R.B., 1976, Deprivation, expectation and threat: effects on salivation in the obese and nonobese. *Physiol. Behav., 17*, 187–193.

Wurtman, R.J. and Fernstrom, J.D., 1975, Control of brain monoamine synthesis by diet and plasma amino acids. *Amer. J. clin. Nutr., 28*, 638–647.

Wyndham, C.H., Williams, C.G. and Loots, H., 1968, Reactions to cold. *J. appl. Physiol., 24*, 282–287.

Wyrwicka, W., 1976, The problem of motivation in feeding behavior. In: D. Novin, W. Wyrwicka and G. Bray (Eds.), *Hunger: Basic Mechanisms and Clinical Implications*, Raven Press, New York, pp. 203–213.

Yang, M.U. and Van Itallie, T.B., 1976, Composition of weight lost during short-term weight reduction. *J. clin. Invest., 58*, 722–730.

Yang, M.U., Wang, J., Pierson, R.M. and Van Itallie, T.B., 1977, Estimation of composition of weight loss in man: a comparison of methods. *J. appl. Physiol., 43*, 331–338.

Young, C.M., 1963, Management of the obese patient. *J. Amer. med. Ass., 186*, 903–909.

Young, C.M., Scanlan, S.S., Topping, C.M., Simko, V. and Lutwak, L., 1971, Frequency of feeding, weight reduction and body composition. *J. Amer. diet. Ass., 59*, 466–472.

Young, R.L., Fuchs, R.J. and Woltjen, M.J., 1976, Chorionic gonadotropin in weight control. *J. Amer. med. Ass., 236*, 2495–2497.

Yudkin, J., 1963, Nutrition and palatability with special reference to obesity, myocardial infarction and other diseases of civilization. *Lancet, i,* 1335–1338.

Yudkin, J., 1974, The low carbohydrate diet. In: W.L. Burland, P.D. Samuel and J. Yudkin (Eds.), *Obesity*, Churchill-Livingstone, Edinburgh, pp. 271–280.

Zuti, W.B. and Golding, L.A., 1973, Equations for estimating percent body fat and body density of active adult males. *Med. Sci. Sports, 5,* 262–266.

Zuti, W.B. and Golding, L.A., 1976, Comparing diet and exercise as weight reduction tools. *Phys. Sportsmed., 4,* 49–53.

Author index

225

232

236

Subject index

240